Pocket Guide to
Electrocardiography

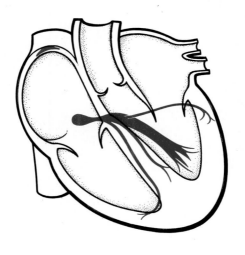

Pocket Guide to
Electrocardiography

Mary Boudreau Conover, R.N., B.S.

Director of Education
Critical Care Conferences
Santa Cruz, California

THIRD EDITION

with **216** illustrations

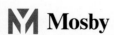 **Mosby**

St. Louis Baltimore Boston Chicago London Madrid
Philadelphia Sydney Toronto

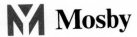

Mosby

Dedicated to Publishing Excellence

Editors: Terry Van Schaik, Timothy M. Griswold
Developmental Editor: Jolynn Gower
Project Manager: Patricia Tannian
Senior Production Editor: Betty Hazelwood
Senior Book Designer: Gail Morey Hudson
Manufacturing Supervisor: Karen Lewis
Cover photograph © Dale Sloat/Phototake, NYC

THIRD EDITION

Copyright © 1994 by Mosby–Year Book, Inc.

Previous editions copyrighted 1986, 1990

Printed in the United States of America
Composition by Graphic World, Inc.
Printing/binding by R. R. Donnelley & Sons Company

Mosby–Year Book, Inc.
11830 Westline Industrial Drive, St. Louis, Missouri 63146

Library of Congress Cataloging in Publication Data

Conover, Mary Boudreau
    Pocket guide to electrocardiography / Mary Boudreau Conover. —
3rd ed.
        p.   cm.
    Includes index.
    ISBN 0-8016-7664-9
    1. Electrocardiography — Handbooks, manuals, etc. 2. Heart —
Diseases — Diagnosis — Handbooks, manuals, etc. 3. Arrhythmia —
Diagnosis — Handbooks, manuals, etc. 4. Heart — Diseases — Nursing —
Handbooks, manuals, etc. I. Title.
    [DNLM: 1. Electrocardiography — handbooks. 2. Electrocardiography —
nurses; instruction. 3. Heart Diseases — diagnosis — handbooks.
4. Arrhythmia — diagnosis — handbooks. WG 39 C753p 1994]
RC683.5.E5C646 1994
616.1'207547 — dc20
DNLM/DLC
for Library of Congress   93-14366
                                                                CIP

93 94 95 96 97 / 9 8 7 6 5 4 3 2 1

Dedicated to
The newlyweds

my daughter
Catherine
and her husband
Thomas C. Boysen, Jr.

Preface

The electrocardiogram has never been so exciting and so informative! New cellular studies and break-through treatment techniques have made this simple, inexpensive tool the bright light of cardiology.

This pocket book of electrocardiography places the diagnosis and treatment of cardiac emergencies at your fingertips. Its concise outline format allows you to carry with you a reference for study of ECG characteristics, mechanisms, clinical implications, and emergency and long-term treatment.

In recent memory the medical community has seen the concepts of cellular electrophysiology revolutionized by the discovery of the patch-clamp technique. With great excitement and hope we have welcomed the technique of radio-frequency ablation for the cure of tachycardias that use accessory pathways; certain types of ventricular tachycardia; and the relief of the rapid rates of symptomatic, refractory atrial fibrillation. We have been encouraged by the medical advances toward the interruption of thrombin generation/formation. Lives have been saved because of the identification of Wellens syndrome, a group of symptoms and ECG signs warning of critical proximal LAD stenosis. The emergency treatment of PSVT has been enhanced and made safer by the use of adenosine. We have learned the dangers of antiarrhythmic drugs and the value of magnesium.

This information has been incorporated into the third edition. Bedside diagnosis of arrhythmias has been added in some cases, and there are four new chapters:

Chapter 4, *Paroxysmal Supraventricular Tachycardia,* offers a side-by-side comparison of the mechanisms of AV nodal reentry tachycardia and circus movement tachycardia using an accessory pathway, the two most common causes of PSVT.

Chapter 11, *Wellens Syndrome,* provides new illustrations and a clear presentation of this important life-saving ECG diagnosis.

Chapter 14, *Acute Pulmonary Embolism,* was added because, although the ECG is not diagnostic, it does provide clues that can save many lives if acted upon promptly with the correct therapy.

Chapter 17, *Emergency Diagnostic Monitoring Leads,* has been added to provide in one place a clear description of leads required for cardiac emergencies.

This compact book provides guidelines for emergency and critical care personnel that results in swift diagnosis and correct response for better patient outcome and professional pride.

Mary Boudreau Conover

Abbreviations

AV	atrioventricular
AVNR	AV nodal reentry
BP	blood pressure
CFX	circumflex (coronary artery)
CMT	circus movement tachycardia (that associated with WPW syndrome)
EPS	electrophysiological studies
LAD	left anterior descending (coronary artery)
LBBB	left bundle branch block
MI	myocardial infarction
PAC	premature atrial complex
PJC	premature junctional complex
PSVT	paroxysmal supraventricular tachycardia
PVC	premature ventricular complex
RBBB	right bundle branch block
RCA	right coronary artery
SVT	supraventricular tachycardia
TdP	torsades de pointes
VA	ventriculoatrial
VF	ventricular fibrillation
VT	ventricular tachycardia

Contents

Principles of Electrocardiography

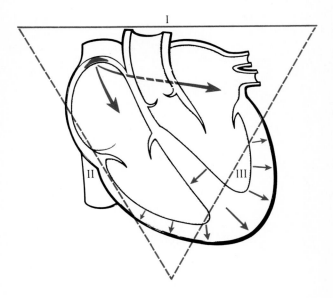

The Electrocardiogram

The electrocardiograph is the instrument that records the electrical activity of the heart, and the electrocardiogram (ECG) is the record of that activity. Electrodes of opposite polarity are placed on the skin at opposite poles of the electrical field; these two electrodes constitute a bipolar lead. One positive electrode and a reference point constitute a unipolar lead. The leads are attached to an amplifier within an oscilloscope or strip recorder. The interpretation of this record is the basis for the ECG diagnosis of arrhythmias.

The 12 Leads

There are six limb leads, three bipolar and three unipolar, and six precordial leads in the standard 12-lead ECG. The precordial leads are unipolar. The limb leads provide information about superior, inferior, right, and left forces; the precordial leads provide information about anterior, posterior, right, and left forces.

The Three Bipolar Limb Leads

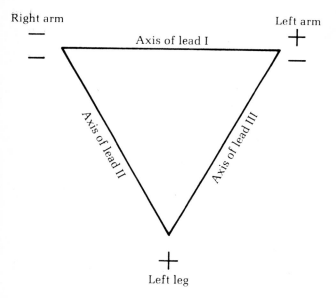

Three bipolar limb leads constitute Einthoven's triangle.

The axis of lead I is from shoulder to shoulder. The negative electrode is on the right arm, and the positive is on the left arm.

The axis of lead II is from the right shoulder to the left leg. The negative electrode is on the right arm, and the positive is on the left leg.

The axis of lead III is from the left shoulder to the left leg. The negative electrode is on the left arm, and the positive is on the left leg.

These electrodes are all about equally distant from the heart; thus the triangle they form is truly equilateral.

The Three Unipolar Limb Leads

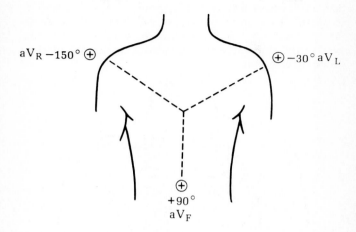

If the two arm electrodes and the left leg electrode are connected to a central terminal through resistances of 5000 ohms each, the sum of the potentials is considered to be zero. The positive exploring electrode is paired with this indifferent reference point (zero) to permit the use of unipolar leads (aV_R, aV_L, or aV_F).

The Precordial Leads

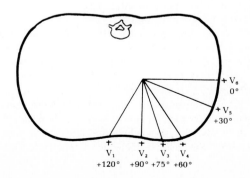

The six principal precordial leads, V_1 to V_6, are unipolar leads whose axes are from the positive electrodes on the chest wall to a zero potential reference point in the center of the electrical field. The electrode positions curve around the thorax over the heart from the right ventricle across the septum to the lateral wall of the left ventricle. Placement of the precordial electrodes is as follows:

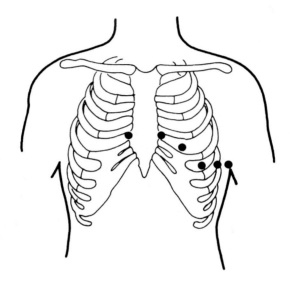

- V_1 and V_2: On either side of the sternum at the fourth interspace
- V_4: Midclavicular line, fifth interspace
- V_3: Midway between V_4 and V_2
- V_5 and V_6: On the same level with V_4 in the anterior and midaxillary lines, respectively

Placement of additional helpful precordial leads is as follows:

- **MCL leads**: These are bipolar chest leads that simulate, for monitoring purposes, the unipolar chest leads. The negative electrode stays in the same position for all of the MCL leads, that is, below the left midclavicle. The position of the positive electrode is identical to that of the unipolar lead to be simulated. For example, to obtain MCL_1, the positive electrode is placed in the fourth interspace right sternal border.

- V_{3R} to V_{6R}: Right precordial leads (unipolar) correspond to left precordial leads V_3 to V_6 (use same chest positions on right chest).

Instant-to-Instant Cardiac Vectors and Electrical Axis

The arrows in the figure below represent the instant-to-instant cardiac vectors, which are numbered in the order of their completion. The sum of all of the cardiac vectors generated during the cardiac cycle is the electrical axis and is represented in this figure by the largest arrow. Even though the currents begin almost simultaneously at the endocardium and proceed to the epicardium in both ventricles, activation of the thicker left ventricular wall takes longer and the currents are stronger. Thus left ventricular forces dominate those of the right ventricle.

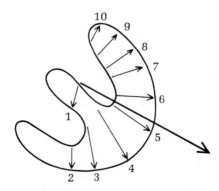

Determination of the P and QRS axis is useful in many clinical settings. In emergency settings, it is used to identify high-risk patients with acute anterior wall infarction, to differentiate between ventricle aberrancy and ventricular ectopy, and to aid in the recognition of pulmonary embolism. The axis can quickly be determined using leads I, II, and aV_F;

for example, I and II are sensitive to the fine movements of the axis in the left upper quadrant, and I and aV$_F$ are used to instantly identify which quadrant the axis is in (normal, right, left, or upper right).

Main Current Flow and the Axis of a Lead

The lead axis is an imaginary line drawn between the two electrodes or between an electrode and a reference point.

When the main current flow is parallel with the axis of a lead, the resulting complex is either the most positive or the most negative deflection of all (Figure 1-1).

When the main current flow is perpendicular to the axis of a lead, an equiphasic deflection is drawn. Note that it does not matter in which direction this current is going; as long as it is perpendicular to the axis of the lead, an equiphasic deflection results.

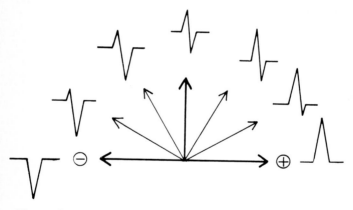

Figure 1-1
A number of mean vectors are combined here to illustrate the possible different complexes. A mean vector that is perpendicular to the lead axis produces an equiphasic deflection. A mean vector on the positive side of the perpendicular and yet not parallel with the lead axis produces a complex that is mostly positive. However, if the mean vector is on the negative side of the perpendicular and yet not parallel with the lead axis, the complex is mostly negative.

An Easy Two-Step Method of Axis Determination

Figure 1-2 is an example of the easy two-step method of axis determination. In the first step, look for an equiphasic deflection; current flow is perpendicular to that lead axis. In this case it is found in aV_R. However, this is incomplete information because the main current flow may be in either direction. So, in the second step, look at the lead whose axis is parallel to this current flow. Current is flowing in the same direction as that lead axis; in this case, lead III. Because the complex in III is negative, current is flowing toward the negative electrode of lead III (left axis deviation [LAD] of −60 degrees).

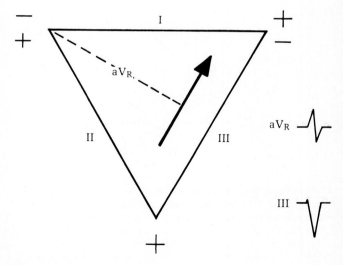

Figure 1-2
Deflections in leads aV_R and III when the axis is −60 degrees (LAD).

Recognizing Axis at a Glance

Normal	Left	Extreme left	Right
−30 to +110°	>0°	>−30°	>+120°

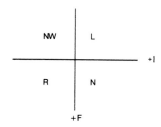

The Quadrant Method of Rapid Axis Determination

The quadrant method uses the axes of leads I and aV_F to divide the thorax into quarters: left (L), normal (N), right (R), and northwest (NW).

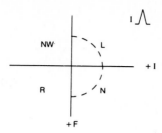

If the complex in lead I is upright, the axis is somewhere in the positive half of lead I.

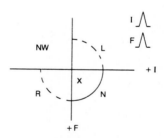

If the complex in lead aV_F is also upright, the axis is in the normal quadrant.

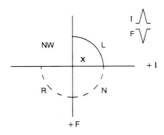

If the complex in lead I is upright and the complex in aV$_F$ is negative, the axis is in the left quadrant. Here is the sole disadvantage of this method: within the left quadrant the axis may be normal (0 to −30 degrees) or abnormal (> −30 degrees). Thus when using this method and left is the quadrant, it is necessary to look at lead II (positive = normal between 0 and −30 degrees; equiphasic = −30 degrees; negative = abnormal > −30 degrees).

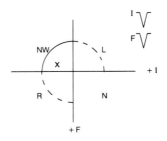

If the complexes in both I and aV$_F$ are negative, the axis is in the NW quadrant ("no man's land").

With this method one can easily see what is meant by "superior" and "inferior" axis. If aV$_F$ is negative, the axis is superior; if aV$_F$ is positive, the axis is inferior.

The Hexaxial Figure

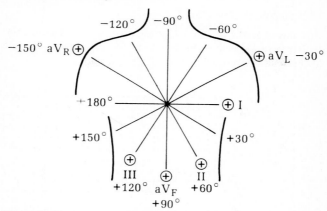

When a more precise determination of axis is needed, the hexaxial figure is used. In the figure above, all of the frontal plane lead axes are drawn through a central point. Each lead axis is at a 30-degree increment with lead I at 0 degrees.

ECG Grid

Time is measured on the horizontal plane of the ECG grid. Each small square is 1 mm in length and represents 0.04 sec. Each larger square is 5 mm long and represents 0.2 sec.

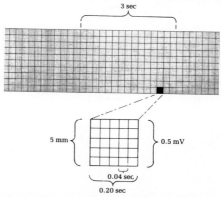

Voltage is measured on the vertical plane, and 1 mV is equal to 10 mm in the standardized ECG.

Step-by-Step Electrical Activation of the Heart Seen in Lead I

The axis of lead I is from left to right (shoulder to shoulder). It therefore is sensitive to the electrical activation of the left atrium and the interventricular (IV) septum.

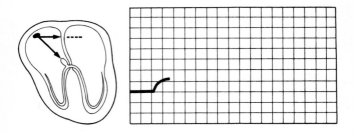

The first half of the P wave is inscribed when the sinus impulse activates the right atrium

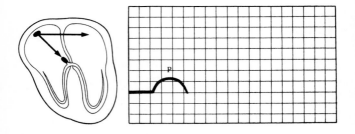

Upon completion of the P wave, the left atrium and atrioventricular (AV) node have been activated

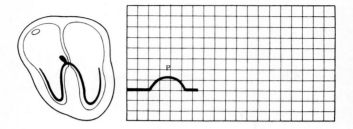

During the isoelectric line after the P wave (the PR segment), the His-Purkinje system is activated

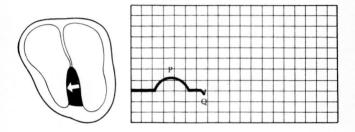

Activation of the IV septum produces a small q wave in lead I

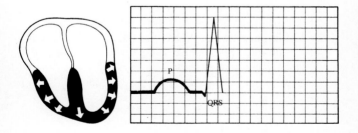

The steep spike of the QRS reflects activation of the walls of the heart; the larger left ventricle dominates

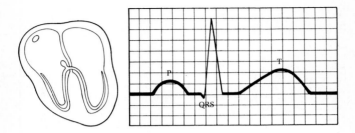

The isoelectric line after the QRS is the ST segment; it is followed by the T wave, which represents ventricular repolarization

ECG Components
P Wave

- Mechanism: Reflects atrial depolarization
- Duration: Not over 0.11 sec
- Amplitude: Not more than 3 mm
- Shape: No notching or peaking
- Polarity:
    1. Positive in I, II, aV_F, V_4 to V_6
    2. Negative in aV_R
    3. Positive, negative, or diphasic in III, aV_L, and V_1 to V_3
    4. If diphasic, the negative component is last and not excessively broad or deep

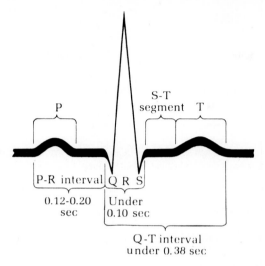

Figure 1-3
Diagrammatic representation of the ECG and its intervals.

■ Clinical significance of abnormalities:
1. Inversion where it should be upright — premature atrial complexes (PACs), retrograde activation from premature junctional complexes (PJCs), or an AV reentry mechanism
2. Increased amplitude — atrial hypertrophy or dilation, usually secondary to AV valve disease, hypertension, cor pulmonale, or congenital heart disease
3. Increased width and notching — left atrial enlargement or diseased atria
4. Diphasic with the negative component excessively wide in II or V_1 — left atrial enlargement
5. Peaking that is taller in I than III — right atrial overload
6. Absent P waves — sinoatrial (SA) block or a junctional rhythm

QRS Complex

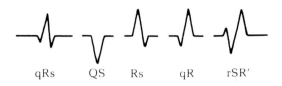

qRs   QS   Rs   qR   rSR′

- Mechanism: Reflects ventricular depolarization
- Duration: Not over 0.10 sec
- Amplitude:
    1. Not less than 5 mm in II, III, aV_F, V_1, and V_6
    2. Not less than 7 mm in V_2 and V_5
    3. Not less than 9 mm in V_3 and V_4
    4. Not over 25 to 30 mm in the precordial leads
- Shape: Positive components are called *R waves*; negative components are either *Q* or *S waves*. A Q wave comes before the first R; an S wave follows the R. *QRS* is a generic term; the exact shape is described by using uppercase and lowercase letters, which indicate the relative sizes of the components.
- Polarity:
    1. Initial forces (septal)
        Narrow q of 1 to 2 mm in V_6, I, and aV_L
        Narrow r in V_1 may normally be absent
    2. Terminal forces (left ventricular)
        S in V_1
        R in V_6
- Clinical significance of abnormalities:
    1. Excessive width reflects intraventricular conduction problems.
    2. Excessive height may indicate hypertrophy or enlargement of the ventricle.
    3. Low voltage may indicate diffuse coronary disease, cardiac failure, pericardial effusion, myxedema, primary amyloidosis, emphysema, obesity, or generalized edema.
    4. The presence or absence of Q waves is judged in the clinical setting.

T Wave

- Mechanism: Reflects ventricular repolarization (phase 3 of the action potential)
- Amplitude: Not more than 5 mm in standard leads and 10 mm in precordial leads
- Shape: Rounded and asymmetrical (notching normal in children)
- Polarity:
    1. Positive in I, II, V_3 to V_6
    2. Negative in aV_R
    3. Positive in aV_L and aV_F, but may be negative if QRS is <5 mm
    4. Varies in III, V_1, and V_2
- Clinical significance of abnormalities:
    1. T wave inversion may indicate diffuse myocardial ischemia or subendocardial infarction, but is not specific.
    2. In the setting of unstable angina, progressive deep symetrical T wave inversion, without loss of R waves in the precordial leads, little or no CK or ST elevation indicates critical proximal left anterior descending (LAD) coronary artery stenosis.
    3. Notching of the T wave, other than in children, may indicate pericarditis.
    4. Sharp and pointed T waves with increased amplitude suggest myocardial infarction or hyperkalemia; also myocardial ischemia and ventricular overload.
    5. T wave alternans may be seen in hypokalemia, hypocalcemia, hypomagnesemia, tachycardia, congestive heart disease, and pericardial disease.

ST Segment

- Mechanism: Represents early stage of ventricular repolarization
- Polarity:
  1. May be elevated slightly (1 mm) in I, II, and III, and 2 mm in the precordial leads
  2. Normally not depressed more than 0.5 mm anywhere
  3. May be depressed as much as 4 mm in precordial leads in young black men (early repolarization syndrome)
- Clinical significance of abnormalities:
  1. Significant displacement — coronary artery disease (marked elevation suggests myocardial infarction, marked depression at rest suggests ischemia or subendocardial infarction, and depression during stress tests suggests occult coronary artery disease). ST depression in approximately 8 leads with slight ST elevation in leads aV_R and V_1 indicates left main and three vessel disease.
  2. Digitalis causes typical depression.
  3. Temporary elevation may result from direct current (DC) cardioversion.

PR Interval

- Mechanism: Represents AV conduction time
- Duration: 0.12 to 0.20 sec
- Clinical significance of abnormalities:
  1. Too short with a normal QRS — Lown-Ganong-Levine syndrome
  2. Too short with a broad QRS — Wolff-Parkinson-White syndrome
  3. Prolonged — AV block or beta blockers

QT Interval

- Mechanism: Represents repolarization time
- Duration: Less than half the preceding RR interval as a general rule. The QT interval is commonly corrected for differences in heart rate by the following formula:

$$QTc = QT/(RR)^{1/2}$$

- Clinical significance of abnormalities: QT lengthening may be idiopathic or caused by drugs (quinidine, procainamide, disopyramide, or amiodarone), electrolyte imbalance (hypokalemia and hypomagnesemia), cerebrovascular disease, hypothermia, or bradycardia. The corrected QT is used in the evaluation of drug effects on ventricular repolarization and the construction of rate-adaptive pacemakers; it may play a role in the prediction of risk after acute myocardial infarction.

U Wave

- Mechanism: Unknown; theories are (1) repolarization of the Purkinje fibers and (2) ventricular relaxation.
- Amplitude: Low voltage
- Polarity: Same as T wave
- Clinical significance of abnormalities:
  1. Hypokalemia (tall U wave)
  2. Reversed polarity in ischemia, left ventricular overload as a result of hypertension, aortic or mitral regurgitation, and left coronary artery disease (at rest)

Calculation of Heart Rate

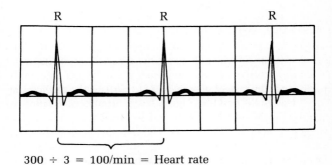

300 ÷ 3 = 100/min = Heart rate

When the rhythm is regular, heart rate can be determined at a glance by counting the large squares between two consecutive R waves and dividing this number into 300.

When the rhythm is irregular, count the R waves in a 6-sec strip and multiply by 10.

Mechanisms of Arrhythmias

The three major classifications for arrhythmogenesis are reentry, altered automaticity, and triggered activity.

Reentry

Reentry is that condition in which a cardiac impulse remains active in a slowly conducting part of the heart and reactivates the heart once the myocardium has repolarized. The current circulates around and around, repeatedly reactivating the fibers in its wake. Three types have been described: anatomical, leading circle, and anisotropic.

Altered Automaticity

Altered automaticity has two subgroups: enhanced normal automaticity and abnormal automaticity. *Enhanced normal automaticity* occurs in the His-Purkinje system as a result of the enhancement of phase 4 depolarization by catecholamines. This type of "slow" ventricular tachycardia is readily suppressed by overdrive pacing. *Abnormal automaticity* is caused by ischemia, infarction, electrolyte derangements, and cardiomyopathy. It may occur anywhere in the heart, even in fibers that in health are not capable of automaticity.

Triggered Activity

Triggered activity is repetitive ectopic firing caused by *afterdepolarizations*, of which there are two types: early and delayed. The early afterdepolarization occurs when the QT interval is prolonged; the triggered activity that results is the mechanism for torsades de pointes. The delayed afterdepolarization is essentially the result of elevated intracellular calcium; the triggered activity that results is the mechanism for the tachycardias of digitalis toxicity. Among other causes of intracellular calcium overload are increased intracellular sodium and decreased extracellular potassium, elevated extracellular calcium, and catecholamines.

Arrhythmias Originating in the Sinus Node

2

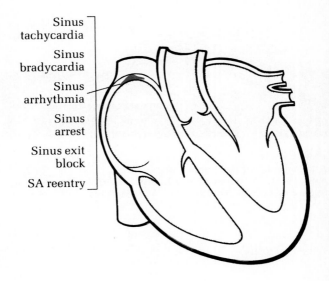

Sinus tachycardia
Sinus bradycardia
Sinus arrhythmia
Sinus arrest
Sinus exit block
SA reentry

The arrhythmias originating in the sinus (or sinoatrial [SA]) node are sinus tachycardia, sinus bradycardia, sinus arrhythmia, SA block, SA nodal reentry, sick sinus syndrome, and sinus arrest.

Anatomy and Physiology

The sinus node is located in the wall of the right atrium, adjacent to the superior vena cava. Figure 2-1 shows that the body of the sinus node blends with perinodal fibers, which in turn blend with atrial tissue. The sinus node has calcium channel action potentials; therefore conduction velocity through the node is normally slow. In a normal sinus rhythm the heart is paced by impulses generated within the sinus node at a rate between 60 and 100 beats/min in the adult according to the needs of the body (autonomic influences).

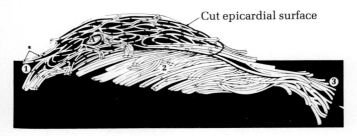
Cut epicardial surface

Figure 2-1
A wax model of the human sinus node.
From Truex RC. In Wellens HJJ, Lie KI, Hanse MJ, editors: *The conduction system of the heart*, Hingham, Mass, 1976, Martinus Nijhoff.

The Normal Sinus P Wave

The normal sinus P wave is upright in leads I, II, aV_F, and V_4 to V_6, and negative in aV_R. The shape of the sinus P wave may change slightly with a shift in pacing sites within the sinus node itself. The normal PR interval is more than 0.12 sec and less than 0.20 sec and may vary slightly with heart rate.

Sinus Tachycardia

Sinus tachycardia is a regular sinus rhythm of more than 100 beats/min. It may be one of the first signs of congestive heart failure, cardiogenic shock, acute pulmonary embolism, or myocardial infarct extension. One should be on the alert for potential problems without waiting for the rate to reach 100 beats/min. In fact, in cases of sepsis, sinus tachycardia is defined as being more than 90 beats/min.

Mechanism

A steepening of phase 4 of the sinus node action potential is the mechanism of sinus tachycardia. This is either (1) the normal response to the demand for increased blood flow, in which case the vagal stimulation is less and the sympathetic stimulation more, resulting in enhanced automaticity in the node, or (2) caused by drugs.

ECG characteristics

II

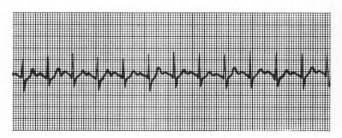

Rate. 100 to 180 beats/min; as high as 200 beats/min during strenuous exercise; this decreases to less than 140 beats/min with age.

Rhythm. Gradual onset and termination.

PR interval. Normal, although the PR may be too long or too short because of other conditions.

QRS complex. Normal, although the QRS may be prolonged as a result of other conditions.

Distinguishing feature. P waves are normal in polarity and occur in front of the QRS. Vagal maneuvers usually cause gradual slowing of the tachycardia, which again accelerates when vagal stimulation is withdrawn.

Causes

- Infancy
- Early childhood
- Exercise
- Emotions
- Fever or pain
- Hypotension
- Thyrotoxicosis
- Anemia
- Hypovolemia
- Pulmonary emboli
- Myocardial ischemia
- Congestive heart failure
- Shock
- Drugs, such as atropine, isoproterenol (Isuprel), quinidine, and epinephrine (Adrenalin), alcohol, nicotine, or caffeine
- Increased sympathetic stimulation

Clinical implications

A physical assessment is indicated because (1) sinus tachycardia is a physiological response to heart failure and (2) in the presence of mitral stenosis or acute ischemic changes, sinus tachycardia may trigger ventricular arrhythmias.

Fever, emotion, pain, and exercise can quickly be evaluated as possible causes. Some patients have an accelerated sinus rate because of a television program, visitors, or frightening or aggravating stimuli around them.

In the complete physical assessment of the patient, listen particularly for a third heart sound, since this, along with sinus tachycardia, is one of the first signs of congestive heart failure. Look for other signs of congestive heart failure.

If the sinus tachycardia is associated with ECG changes (see p. 176), dyspnea, and sudden chest pain, acute pulmonary embolism should be suspected and the physician notified. The ECG plus echocardiographic signs are diagnostic of acute pulmonary embolism.

A 12-lead ECG should be obtained to ascertain the presence of infarct extension.

Bedside diagnosis

- Regular pulse
- Normal neck vein pulsation
- Constant systolic blood pressure
- Constant intensity of first heart sound
- Gradual and temporary slowing of heart rate with vagal maneuvers

Rhythm variations

Sinus tachycardias vary only if they are part of a bradycardia-tachycardia syndrome or because of associated conditions, such as atrioventricular (AV) block, bundle branch block (BBB), premature ventricular complexes (PVCs), or premature atrial complexes (PACs).

Differential diagnosis

The P waves in the atrial tachycardia of digitalis toxicity (rate: 130-250) are identical in shape to those of sinus tachycardia. The clinical setting and sometimes the heart rate help to differentiate.

Treatment

None, although a clinical assessment is indicated and the cause of the sinus tachycardia is treated or eliminated (e.g., alcohol, caffeine, tobacco, nose drops containing sympathomimetic agents).

Sinus Bradycardia

Sinus bradycardia is a regular sinus rhythm of less than 60 beats/min.

Mechanism

Sinus bradycardia is either (1) the normal response to decreased demand for blood flow, in which case the vagal stimulation is more and the sympathetic stimulation less, resulting in decreased automaticity in the SA node, such as during sleep or in trained athletes or (2) the result of increased vagal tone in myocardial infarction (MI) and may or may not be accompanied by hypotension. Sinus bradycardia occurs as part of the sick sinus syndrome.

ECG characteristics

II

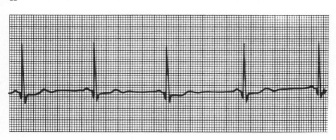

Rate.   < 60 beats/min.
Rhythm.   Regular.
PR interval.   Normal, although the PR may be too long or too short because of other conditions. All of the P waves are the same shape and are upright in leads I, II, aV_F, and V_4 to V_6.
QRS complex.   Normal, although the QRS may be prolonged as a result of other conditions.
Distinguishing features.   Rate, rhythm, and uniform shape of the P waves. The slow rate is quickly diagnosed because there are more than 5 large squares between R waves.

Causes

- Sleep
- Athletic heart
- Increased vagal tone or decreased sympathetic tone
- Meningitis
- Increased intracranial pressure
- Cervical or mediastinal tumor
- Hypoxia
- Myxedema
- Hypothermia
- Fibrodegenerative changes
- Gram-negative sepsis
- Mental depression
- Eye surgery
- Coronary arteriography
- Vomiting and vasovagal syncope

Clinical implications

Sinus bradycardia is noted as a transient event during acute MI (more so during inferior than anterior MI) and is beneficial unless accompanied by hemodynamic deterioration or other arrhythmias. If the bradycardia is profound or associated with other arrhythmias, hemodynamic compromise may occur, which is the only reason for intervention.

Rhythm variations

Sinus bradycardias vary only if they are part of a bradycardia-tachycardia syndrome or because of associated conditions, such as AV block, bundle branch block, PVCs, or PACs. The diagnosis of sinus bradycardia is made because of the underlying rhythm.

Differential diagnosis

Bigeminal nonconducted PACs.

Treatment

Usually none, unless there is hemodynamic compromise, in which case atropine (0.5 mg IV and repeated as necessary) may be used.

Sinus Arrhythmia

Sinus arrhythmia is an irregular sinus rhythm in which the cycle lengths vary so that the difference between the shortest PP interval and the longest PP interval is >0.12 sec.

Mechanism

Sinus arrhythmia has two types: respiratory and nonrespiratory. The *respiratory* form is prominent in the young, is the normal response of the heart to respiration, and is especially marked in children. The rate increases with inspiration (reflex inhibition of vagal tone) and decreases with expiration. The *nonrespiratory* form may be related to digitalis toxicity.

ECG characteristics

II

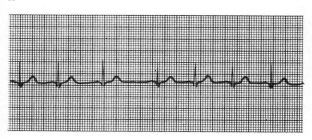

Rate.   Varies with respiration (faster with inspiration, slower with expiration).

Rhythm.   Irregular.

PR interval.   Normal, although the PR may be too long or too short because of other conditions. All of the P waves are the same shape and are upright in leads I, II, aV_F, and V_4 to V_6.

QRS complex.   Normal, although the QRS may be prolonged as a result of other conditions.

Distinguishing features.   Varying rate; cyclical, irregular rhythm; and uniform shape of the P waves.

Causes

- Normal respiratory pattern
- Digitalis toxicity

Clinical implications

The respiratory form of sinus arrhythmia is benign; the nonrespiratory form may be a sign of digitalis toxicity.

There may be hemodynamic compromise during the slower phase of this rhythm, especially if a junctional escape beat does not appear.

During the early phase of acute MI, loss of heart rate variability is a risk factor for sudden cardiac death.

Differential diagnosis

SA nodal reentry may resemble sinus arrhythmia because the P waves are the same as normal sinus P waves in both rhythms. However, in SA reentry the transition to a faster rate is abrupt and not related to respiration.

Treatment

Usually none; increasing the heart rate with exercise helps; symptomatic patients are treated for sinus bradycardia.

Sick Sinus Syndrome

Sick sinus syndrome (SSS) is a clinical syndrome manifesting abnormal sinus nodal function as a result of a wide range of cellular physiological abnormalities, associated with derangement in SA nodal impulse formation, transmission, and conduction.

Mechanism

SSS occurs more frequently in inferior than in anterior MI because of ischemia of the AV node, stimulation of Bezold-Jarisch reflexes*, or release of potassium and adenosine from the ischemic cells. Sinus node artery disease and atrial disease also may be factors. Pediatric cardiac surgery or insertion of atrial cannulae may damage the sinus node and later cause SSS.

Abnormalities in both sinus node automaticity and SA conduction are responsible for the long sinus or atrial pauses in SSS.

---

*When ischemia stimulates the afferent nerves adjacent to the AV node, the resulting increased vagal tone produces sinus bradycardia, hypotension, and sometimes heart block.

ECG characteristics

II

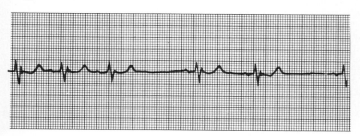

Rate.   Too fast or too slow.

Rhythm.   Irregular.

PR interval.   May be abnormal.

QRS complex.   Normal, although the QRS may be prolonged because of other conditions.

Distinguishing features.   Any of the following arrhythmias may be present and associated with syncope:

1. Marked, symptomatic, or inappropriate sinus bradycardia or sinus arrhythmia
2. SA exit block
3. Sinus pauses or sinus arrest
4. Chronic atrial tachycardia with a slow ventricular response
5. Bradycardia-tachycardia
6. Sinus bradycardia with recurring atrial fibrillation (thought to be preterminal)

The diagnosis can be made if a Stokes-Adams episode occurs in association with supraventricular arrhythmias.

Causes

- Ischemic disease
- Surgical injury
- Inflammatory disease
- Amyloidosis
- Collagen disease
- Metastatic disease
- Idiopathic

Clinical implications

Take a careful history to see if a definable underlying cause exists, such as digitalis, beta blockers, calcium channel blockers, or (occasionally) diuretics.

Notify the physician and closely monitor the patient.

Be ready for emergency supportive measures. The patient may be a candidate for a permanent pacemaker and may require temporary emergency pacing if there is hemodynamic compromise and the sinus node has not responded to treatment.

Rhythm variations

Many variations exist and include the following:

II

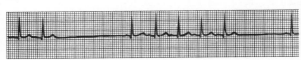

- SSS with Type II second-degree SA block

V₁

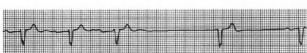

- SSS in the form of a bradycardia-tachycardia syndrome

II

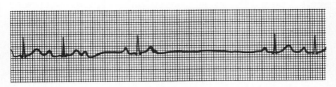

- SSS with inappropriate overdrive supression after an early PAC (in the T wave before the pause)

Treatment

Studies have shown that patients with SSS are less likely to develop atrial fibrillation when they are treated with AV synchronous pacemakers (DDD or AAI pacemaker). Before a pacemaker is inserted, ensure that no drugs at all have been given for several days; the arrhythmia may be drug related. Anticoagulation is necessary in spite of pacemaker therapy.

 ## SA Exit Block

SA exit block is a defect in conduction from the sinus node to atrial tissue.

Mechanism

The sinus impulses are generated, but not all of them are conducted, resulting in intermittently absent P waves.

ECG characteristics

V₁

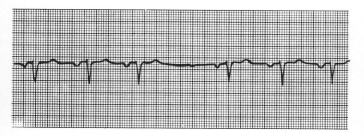

Type I (Wenckebach) SA block. PP intervals shorten until a P wave is dropped; pauses are less than twice the shortest cycle (a longer strip would show group beating).

II

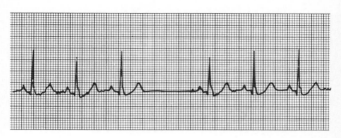

Type II SA block.   PP intervals are an exact multiple of the sinus cycle and are regular and fixed before and after the dropped P wave.

Causes

- Excessive vagal stimulation
- Myocardial infarction
- Potassium derangements
- Acute myocarditis
- Atrial fibrosis
- Drugs such as sympatholytics, beta blockers, calcium channel blockers, classes IA and IC antiarrhythmic drugs, and acetylcholine

Clinical implications

The diagnosis is made because of a pause in the place of a normal sinus P wave.

SA exit block is usually transient.

There may be hemodynamic compromise if the pauses are too long. The patient should be evaluated for decreased blood pressure, confusion, or increased number of ventricular ectopics, since these are the only reason for treating this arrhythmia.

The physician should be notified, because SA block is a possible manifestation of underlying heart disease. A pacemaker may be indicated if there is hemodynamic compromise and the sinus node has not responded to treatment.

Differential diagnosis

Nonconducted PACs are far more common than SA block and should be suspected first when unexpected pauses occur in the ECG. Usually the P' wave can be seen distorting the T wave before the pause. The diagnosis of sinus arrest can be made after ruling out nonconducted PACs and SA block.

Treatment

None, if there is no hemodynamic compromise. Otherwise, therapy is that of sinus bradycardia.

 # Sinus Arrest or Sinus Pause

Sinus arrest or sinus pause is a failure of impulse formation in the sinus node.

Mechanism

This is a defect in impulse formation. There is a marked depression in sinus node activity.

ECG characteristics

V_1

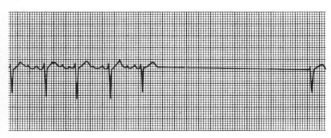

    Rate.   Normal, but varies because of pauses.

    Rhythm.   Underlying rhythm regular with pauses that have no numerical relationship to the basic rhythm.

    PR interval.   Normal and fixed, unless associated with prolonged AV conduction.

    QRS complex.   Normal, although the QRS may be prolonged because of other conditions.

Distinguishing features.   Abrupt interruption of the sinus rhythm. PP interval of the pause is not a multiple of the sinus cycle as in type II SA block. The diagnosis is impossible to make with certainty on the surface ECG.

Causes

- Acute MI involving the sinus node
- Degenerative fibrosis
- Digitalis toxicity
- Stroke
- Excessive vagal tone

Clinical implications

Not clinically significant as long as there are junctional escape beats during excessive pauses in sinus nodal activity.

The patient should be evaluated for decreased blood pressure, confusion, or increased number of ventricular ectopics, since these are the only reasons for treating this arrhythmia.

Differential diagnosis

Nonconducted PACs are far more common and are always suspected first. Usually the P′ wave can be seen distorting the T wave before the pause. The diagnosis of sinus arrest can be made after ruling out nonconducted PACs and SA block.

Treatment

None, if there is no hemodynamic compromise. Otherwise, treatment is that of sinus bradycardia.

SA Nodal Reentry

SA nodal reentry is one of the less common causes of PSVT (5% to 10%).

Mechanism

The SA node itself is the perfect type of tissue to support a reentry circuit, which can be initiated by a sinus impulse that does not exit the sinus node uniformly, leaving a nonrefractory pathway by which the impulse can return into the SA node and establish a reentry circuit. This reentry mechanism does not depend on slow conduction in the atria; the slow conduction necessary to a reentry circuit occurs as the impulse passes through the sinus node.

ECG characteristics

V₁

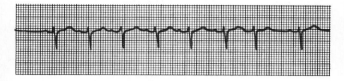

Rate.   80 to 200 beats/min (average 130-140 beats/min).

Rhythm.   PSVT.

PR interval.   Usually short; related to the rate of the tachycardia; P waves are similar or identical in shape to normal sinus P waves. AV block may exist without influencing the tachycardia.

QRS complex.   Normal, although the QRS may be prolonged as a result of other conditions.

Distinguishing features.   Heart rate suddenly accelerates; tachycardia ends abruptly; rhythm of the tachycardia usually regular; normal sinus P waves; Wenckebach AV conduction common; vagal maneuvers can slow and then abruptly terminate the tachycardia.

Causes

- Ischemia
- Cardiomyopathy

Clinical implications

Usually none; patients may not even notice the tachycardia.

Patients may have a higher incidence of heart disease than those with other forms of PSVT

In some patients, SA nodal reentry may be the mechanism in so-called "anxiety-related sinus tachycardia."

Differential diagnosis

Sinus arrhythmia.

Treatment

None, unless the patient is symptomatic; if that is the case, propranolol, verapamil, or digitalis may terminate the tachycardia and prevent recurrences.

Hypersensitive Carotid Sinus Syndrome

Cardioinhibitory carotid sinus hypersensitivity is ventricular asystole of more than 3 seconds during carotid sinus stimulation.

    Vasodepressor carotid sinus hypersensitivity is a decrease in systolic blood pressure of 50 mm Hg or more without associated cardiac slowing.

Mechanism

The mechanism is not known. Suspected mechanisms are (1) excessive resting vagal tone, (2) excessive acetylcholine, (3) hypersensitive baroreflex, (4) inadequate cholinesterase, and (5) concomitant sympathetic withdrawal.

ECG characteristics

Atrial standstill because of sinus arrest or SA exit block coupled with failure of junctional or ventricular escape beats.

Causes

- Coronary artery disease
- Tight collar, head turning, or neck tension (reduces blood flow through the vertebral arteries

Treatment

Note: Nonsymptomatic patients are not treated. The syndrome may be enhanced by drugs like digitalis, alphamethyldopa, clonidine, and propranolol. Severe cases may require radiation therapy or surgical denervation of the carotid sinus.

    Cardioinhibitory form: Generally, atropine and ventricular pacing with or without atrial pacing for symptomatic patients.

    Vasodepressor form: Atropine does not prevent decrease in systemic blood pressure; vasodepression may cause continued syncope even after pacemaker implantation. Elastic support hose and sodium-retaining drugs may be helpful.

Atrial and Junctional Beats and Rhythms

3

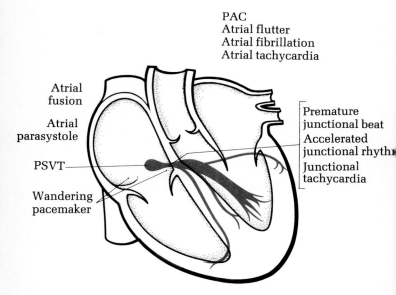

PAC
Atrial flutter
Atrial fibrillation
Atrial tachycardia

Atrial fusion

Atrial parasystole

PSVT

Wandering pacemaker

Premature junctional beat
Accelerated junctional rhythm
Junctional tachycardia

This chapter is divided into two main sections: Atrial Beats and Rhythms and Junctional Beats and Rhythms. Atrial fusion beats and atrial parasystole are covered also. Paroxysmal supraventricular tachycardia is covered in Chapter 4.

Atrial Beats and Rhythms

Atrial beats and rhythms consist of premature atrial complexes (PACs), atrial tachycardia, atrial fibrillation, and atrial flutter. Premature sinus beats may occur also, but they are not commonly recognized.

Premature Atrial Complexes

PACs are premature atrial beats that originate within the atria but outside of the sinus node. The resulting ECG deflection is called a P' (P prime) wave, meaning a secondary P wave.

Mechanism

PACs are the result of abnormal automaticity or triggered activity. The mechanisms of AV conduction and pauses after PACs are described here.

AV conduction. The five possible mechanisms of AV conduction are the following:

1. Normal conduction.
2. Nonconduction (blocked PAC).
3. Conduction with bundle branch block, hemiblock (aberrant ventricular conduction), or both.
4. Conduction solely down the slow intranodal pathway, leaving the fast intranodal pathway free for retrograde conduction and setting the stage for an AV nodal reentry circuit and PSVT.
5. In patients with accessory pathways, a PAC may conduct down the AV node to the ventricles and return to the atria via the accessory pathway, setting up an AV reentry circuit and PSVT.

The post-PAC pause. The pause after a PAC is determined by several factors:

1. The PAC invades a nonrefractory sinus node and resets it, causing the next expected sinus P wave to be on time *if measured from the PAC* but earlier than it would have been if the sinus node had not been prematurely activated (a noncompensatory pause).
2. The premature activation of the sinus node may depress its automaticity (overdrive suppression) and cause the next sinus P wave to be late.
3. Less commonly, the sinus node is refractory to stimulation from the PAC and is neither reset nor suppressed (the full compensatory pause).
4. Rarely, the PAC may be interpolated.

ECG characteristics

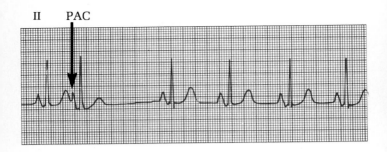

Rate.   That of the underlying rhythm.

Rhythm.   Irregular, resulting from PACs (underlying rhythm may be regular).

PR interval.   The P'-R interval may be the same as that of the sinus rhythm, or it may be prolonged as a result of conduction down the slow AV nodal pathway; or the PAC may not be conducted to the ventricles (a blocked PAC).

QRS complex.   Normal, although the QRS may be prolonged as a result of bundle branch block (BBB) or aberrancy (a functional BBB caused by a shortening of the cycle length).

Distinguishing features.   The diagnosis is made because of an irregular rhythm and premature, ectopic-looking P waves, which may be clearly visible or may distort T waves.

Causes

- Emotion
- Nicotine
- Alcohol
- Caffeine
- Infection or inflammation
- Myocardial ischemia
- Atrial dilation or hypertrophy resulting from mitral stenosis or atrial septal defect
- Electrolyte imbalance
- Hypoxia
- Digitalis toxicity

Clinical implications

In the setting of acute myocardial infarction, PACs are frequently a result of catecholamines released secondary to apprehension and pain. Once the patient is reassured and given morphine, the PACs often disappear. Also, since many people are smokers and come in with hypoxia (a cause of atrial ectopy), oxygen effectively treats the PACs.

Although PACs are not life-threatening, in association with acute myocardial infarction they warn of congestive heart failure, electrolyte imbalance, or both. PACs may precipitate atrial flutter, atrial fibrillation, or PSVT. The resulting fall in cardiac output may cause further myocardial damage and may precipitate ventricular tachycardia. If bigeminal nonconducted PACs develop, the resulting bradycardia may be profound and may cause hemodynamic deterioration, even in the otherwise healthy heart.

Rhythm variations

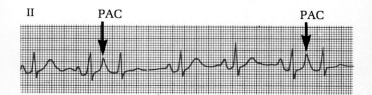

PACs hidden in T waves

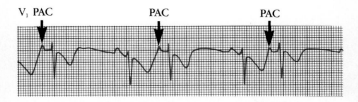

Bigeminal PACs

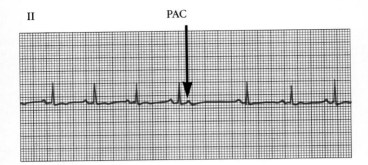

Nonconducted PAC

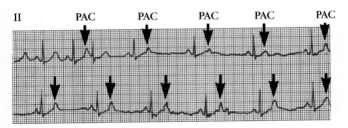

Bigeminal nonconducted PACs

Differential diagnosis

Sinus arrest or SA block. Nonconducted PACs are statistically far more common and can usually be spotted distorting the T wave.

Treatment

PACs are not treated. If they are causing the onset of PSVT, dietary measures may help (more potassium, less caffeine).

 Atrial Tachycardia

Atrial tachycardia is divided into three types according to mechanism: abnormal automaticity, triggered activity, and intraatrial reentry.

Mechanisms

At the cellular level, abnormal automaticity is the result of a loss of negativity, such as occurs with ischemia or injury to the cell. Triggered activity secondary to digitalis excess is caused by delayed afterdepolarizations, which are in turn the result of excess calcium in the cell. Atrial reentry may be caused by a microreentry circuit within the atria. Reports of its occurrence are published infrequently.

ECG characteristics

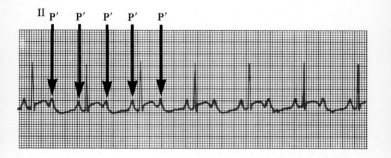

Rate. Digitalis induced: 130 to 250 beats/min (atrial). Abnormal automaticity: < 200 beats/min (atrial). Reentry: 130 to 180 beats/min (atrial). The ventricular rate depends on the AV conduction ratio.

Rhythm. May be regular or irregular because of competing pacemaker sites or because of ventriculophasic PP intervals (i.e., in 2:1 block, PP intervals embracing the QRS may be shorter than PP intervals without a QRS).

PR interval. P'R interval is influenced by the rate of the atria.

QRS complex. Normal, although the QRS may be prolonged because of functional or pathological BBB.

Distinguishing features. P wave polarity, rate, and rhythm. In digitalis toxicity the P wave axis is superior-inferior (positive in lead II and similar in shape to the sinus P wave). There may be ventriculophasic PP intervals in the setting of digitalis toxicity; that is, in 2:1 block the PP interval that contains the QRS is shorter than the one that does not.

Causes

- Myocardial infarction
- Coronary artery disease
- Chronic lung disease
- Metabolic derangements (such as would occur with acute alcohol ingestion)
- Digitalis toxicity (potassium depletion may precipitate this arrhythmia)

Clinical implications

The underlying cardiovascular status and the mechanism of the atrial tachycardia determine the signs, symptoms, and prognosis.

Atrial tachycardia caused by digitalis toxicity: in a well-known study by Driefus, if the tachycardia was caused by digitalis toxicity, failure to discontinue the drug was shown to carry a mortality of 100%. The patient is monitored carefully, and the physical assessment determines therapy.

Chronic atrial tachycardia: this type of atrial tachycardia is uncommon and usually is seen in children and young adults. Progressive cardiac dilation and congestive heart failure may result.

Bedside diagnosis

- Regular pulse
- Normal neck vein pulsation
- Constant systolic BP
- Constant intensity of first heart sound
- Carotid sinus massage causes temporary slowing of ventricular rate or has no effect (nonparoxysmal type)

Variations

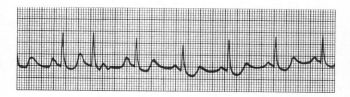

Atrial tachycardia with 4:3 AV Wenckebach conduction and with 2:1 AV conduction (the first two P waves are conducted with PR intervals of 0.12 sec and 0.20 sec; the third P wave is not conducted; the remainder of the tracing shows 2:1 conduction)

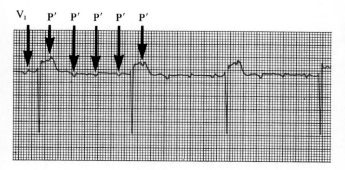

Atrial tachycardia with 4:1 AV conduction (other conduction ratios are possible also)

Differential diagnosis

When abnormal automaticity is the mechanism, the P′ wave differs in contour from the sinus P wave and the rate is less than 200 beats/min.

In atrial tachycardia seen in digitalis toxicity, the P′ wave is almost identical in shape to the sinus P wave because the focus is close to the sinus node, and the rate may be as high as 250 beats/min. The initiating P′ wave is identical to the subsequent ones in both of these atrial tachycardias.

In the reentrant type of atrial tachycardia, the initiating P′ is different from subsequent ones. Vagal maneuvers do not terminate these tachycardias, although they may produce AV block.

Treatment

Atrial tachycardia caused by digitalis toxicity: the digitalis is discontinued, and potassium chloride is given orally or intravenously. The patient should be protected from sympathetic stimulation (complete bed rest). If there is hemodynamic deterioration, digitalis antibody may be used. If Dilantin is used, a pacemaker may be necessary also. Often simply discontinuing the digitalis will resolve the rhythm.

Chronic atrial tachycardia: radio-frequency catheter ablation has been shown to be safe and effective in patients refractory to antiarrhythmia drugs. Surgical excision of the focus has been used in the past.

 Multifocal (Chaotic) Atrial Tachycardia
ECG characteristics

V_1

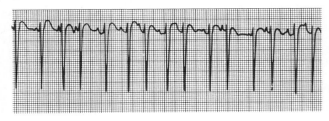

Rate.   100 to 130 beats/min.
Rhythm.   Irregular.
PR interval.   May or may not be normal. P′-R intervals may vary.
QRS complex.   Normal, although it may be broad as a result of BBB.
Distinguishing features.   P′ waves of usually three different shapes and an irregular rhythm, with most P waves conducted to the ventricles.

Mechanism

The mechanism is thought to be triggered activity caused by delayed afterdepolarizations.

Causes

- Chronic pulmonary disease
- Hypoxia
- Electrolyte derangement

Clinical implications

This arrhythmia carries a high mortality because of the clinical implications of the primary disease (usually chronic obstructive pulmonary disease and congestive heart failure in an older patient).

Differential diagnosis

Atrial fibrillation (a 12-lead ECG usually reveals the P waves of the multifocal atrial tachycardia).

Treatment

Chaotic atrial tachycardia is a difficult arrhythmia to treat. Treatment is that of the underlying disease, which may be cardiac, pulmonary, metabolic, or infection. Reports indicate that it may respond to calcium channel blockers, such as verapamil and magnesium sulfate, or to potassium and magnesium. Amiodarone has been helpful also.

Atrial Flutter

Atrial flutter is a rapid and regular atrial rhythm. Usually the atrial rate is 300 beats/min, but it may range from 230 to 430 beats/min and is divided into type I and type II according to rate. *Flutter-fibrillation* has a variable contour and rate, which is faster than atrial flutter, and may in fact be dissimilar atrial rhythms.

Mechanism

The mechanism of atrial flutter is a single reentry circuit within the right atrium. Prolonged atrial conduction time is a predisposing factor.

ECG characteristics

II

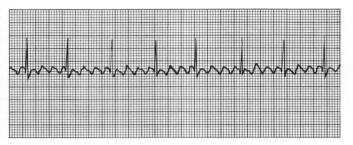

Rate

Atrial: In type I (classical) the atrial rate ranges from 230 to 350 beats/min; in type II the range is from 340 to 430 beats/min.

Ventricular: Usually 150 to 170 beats/min because of the common 2:1 AV conduction ratio; in the absence of drugs a significantly slower ventricular rate suggests abnormal AV conduction.

Rhythm.   Atrial rhythm is regular; ventricular rhythm depends on the AV conduction pattern (regular with a fixed conduction ratio; group beating with Wenckebach conduction; and irregular when AV conduction varies).

P'R interval.   0.26 to 0.46 sec.

QRS complex.   Normal unless functional or pathological BBB is present.

AV conduction.   Usually an even number, such as 2:1, 4:1, 6:1, but may alternate between 2:1 at the top of the AV node and 3:2 Wenckebach at the bottom of the AV node, resulting in group beating of the ventricular rhythm.

Distinguishing features.   Regular sawtooth pattern in II, III, aV_F; sharp positive P' waves in V_1; lack of isoelectric interval between flutter waves (implies continuous electrical activity of the reentry circuit); normal QRS complexes.

Causes

- Any form of heart disease
- Acute illness
- Thyrotoxicosis
- Alcoholism
- Pericarditis
- Atrial dilation
- Pulmonary emboli
- Mitral or tricuspid valve stenosis or regurgitation
- Chronic ventricular failure

Clinical implications

Paroxysmal atrial flutter is seen in normal hearts; chronic atrial flutter is more common in patients over 40 years of age with myocardial ischemia, cardiomyopathy, or rheumatic heart disease.

If the onset is sudden, notify the physician and prepare to administer digitalis or perform electrical cardioversion.

In children, continued episodes are associated with the possibility of sudden death.

Caution: Exercise can double the ventricular rate (sympathetic tone increases; vagal tone decreases).

Bedside diagnosis

- Regular pulse with 2:1 conduction
- Irregular pulse with variable conduction
- Flutter waves in the neck veins
- Constant systolic BP with regular pulse
- Changing systolic BP with irregular pulse
- Constant intensity of first heart sound
- Carotid sinus massage causes temporary slowing of ventricular rate, conversion into atrial fibrillation, or no effect

Rhythm variations

II

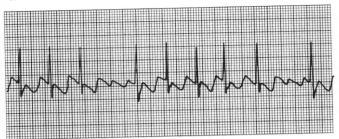

Atrial flutter with 2:1 and 4:1 AV conduction ratios

II

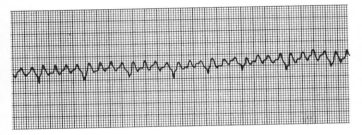

Atrial flutter with 4:1 and 3:1 conduction ratios

II

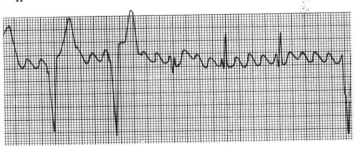

Atrial flutter with AV dissociation (an accelerated idio-ventricular rhythm with one fusion and two capture beats)

Differential diagnosis

When the conduction ratio is 2:1, atrial flutter often is mistaken for sinus tachycardia of 140 to 175 beats/min. The ventricular rate makes one suspicious of a hidden flutter wave, and often the onset of the R wave is distorted by the flutter wave.

Treatment

1. Synchronous direct current (DC) cardioversion (usually < 50 joules).
2. Rapid atrial pacing with an esophageal catheter or right atrial catheter (for type I atrial flutter).
3. If unsuccessful, digitalis with a beta blocker or calcium channel blocker (to slow the ventricular rate).
4. Low-dose amiodarone (to prevent recurrence).

   Note: Studies have shown that radio-frequency ablation of a relatively small area of endocardium in the right atrium terminates and prevents recurrence of atrial flutter.

Atrial Fibrillation

Atrial fibrillation is an arrhythmia characterized by erratic depolarization of the atria.

Mechanism

Atrial fibrillation is generated and maintained by one or more rapidly firing ectopic foci, from which emanate multiple waves of electrical current forming random reentry circuits.

ECG characteristics

V$_1$

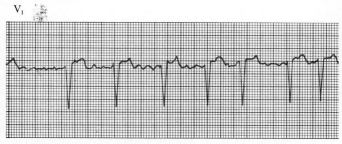

   Rate (ventricular).   Uncontrolled, 100 to 180 beats/min; controlled (drug-induced prolongation of AV conduction), 70 to 80 beats/min.

Rhythm.   Irregular.

PR interval.   Absent P waves.

QRS complex.   Normal unless associated with BBB.

Distinguishing features.   Absent P waves and irregular ventricular response.

Causes

- Mitral valve disease
- Myocardial infarction (after first 24 hours secondary to pericarditis or heart failure)
- Ischemic heart disease
- Rheumatic heart disease
- Hypertension
- Thyrotoxicosis
- Increasing left atrial size in elderly patients
- Seen in the absence of any apparent disease
- Associated with Wolff-Parkinson-White syndrome

Clinical implications

Atrial fibrillation may be intermittent or chronic, which carries the greater risk. Approximately 2% of U.S. population over 60 years of age and 4% over 70 years have atrial fibrillation. Most affected individuals have underlying heart disease, with prolonged atrial conduction time or atrial enlargement. In recent-onset atrial fibrillation, thyrotoxicosis is considered.

The inefficient movement of blood in the atria predisposes the patient to the formation of emboli; this risk is especially high in patients with rheumatic heart disease (RHD) (17 times greater than without RHD). In the hemodynamically stable patient, the rhythm may spontaneously convert within 2 to 3 hours.

The physician should be notified of sudden-onset atrial fibrillation. If conversion is not spontaneous, prepare for cardioversion and evaluate for shock and myocardial ischemia (anginal chest pain, ST segment depressions or elevations, new Q waves, inverted T waves).

In patients with chronic atrial fibrillation, evaluate for the following:

1. Digitalis toxicity, if applicable (QRS regularity, group beating, ventricular ectopics, or symptoms such as visual complaints, and psuedodementia)

2. Congestive heart failure (difficult breathing, pedal edema, and crackles at lung bases)

Bedside diagnosis

- Irregular pulse
- Irregular neck vein pulsation
- Changing systolic blood pressure
- Changing intensity of first heart sound
- Carotid sinus massage causes temporary slowing of ventricular rate or has no effect

Rhythm variations

III

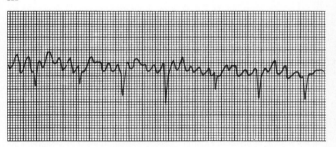

Coarse atrial fibrillation with signs of digitalis toxicity (regularization of the ventricular response)

II

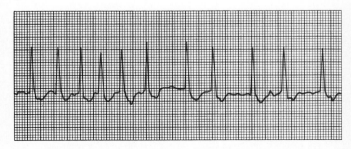

Fine atrial fibrillation with uncontrolled ventricular response

V₁

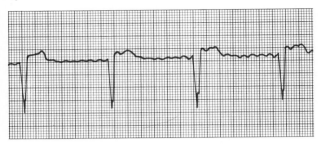

Atrial fibrillation with complete AV block

II

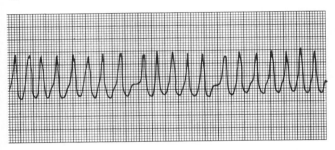

Atrial fibrillation with conduction over an accessory pathway

Differential diagnosis

Uncontrolled atrial fibrillation may occasionally resemble sinus tachycardia when the fibrillatory line contains components that resemble P waves. Remember that in sinus tachycardia there is a P wave of identical shape in front of *every* QRS.

Treatment

1. Slow the ventricular response (common drugs are digoxin, beta adrenergic antagonists, and calcium antagonists). Caution: When an accessory pathway is present, these drugs should not be given.
2. Convert the atria to sinus rhythm (common drugs are class IA, class IC, and amiodarone).

3. Electrical cardioversion is considered if drug therapy is not effective, and it is the treatment of choice in sudden-onset atrial fibrillation with hemodynamic decomposition.
4. An anticoagulant (warfarin) is used to reduce risk of stroke.
5. When atrial fibrillation develops in a patient with an accessory pathway (WPW syndrome), procainamide is given to block the accessory pathway. If this is not successful, emergency DC cardioversion is used. Such patients must be referred for radio-frequency ablation of their accessory pathway, which is a cure.

Junctional Beats and Rhythms

Junctional beats and rhythms consist of premature junctional complexes (PJCs), accelerated junctional rhythms, junctional tachycardia, junctional escape beats, and junctional escape rhythms.

Mechanism

PJCs, accelerated junctional rhythms, and junctional tachycardia are the result of triggered activity or altered automaticity in the bundle of His. The focus is usually the same as that of the primary junctional escape focus, that is, the proximal bundle of His (lower AV node). Junctional escape mechanisms are the normal response of the heart to bradycardia. The mechanism of the accelerated junctional rhythm (rate, 62-99 beats/min) and junctional tachycardia (rate, 100-140 beats/min) is the same; they traditionally are divided according to rate and may be secondary to digitalis toxicity, ischemia, or catecholamines. When the ectopic focus discharges, the current may be blocked in the retrograde direction into the atria. This is called an *idiojunctional rhythm* (i.e., AV dissociation exists). When digitalis is involved, there is usually AV dissociation. If retrograde conduction is not blocked, there will be a retrograde P′ wave that may be before, during (not seen), or after the QRS complex, depending on the relative speeds of anterograde and retrograde conduction and the location of the ectopic focus in the bundle of His.

The mechanism of junctional escape beats and rhythms is the emergence of the normal automaticity of the bundle of His in response to excessively long pauses in the cardiac rhythm. It is a protective mechanism.

ECG characteristics

Rate.   That of the underlying rhythm (sinus or junctional).

Rhythm.   PJCs cause irregularity; junctional rhythms are regular.

PR interval.   Does not apply. The P wave is retrograde in some cases, and there is AV dissociation in others.

QRS complex.   Narrow unless there is also bundle branch block.

Distinguishing features.   QRS complex identical to sinus conducted ones. If there is retrograde conduction to the atria, the P′ wave is negative in II, III, and aV$_F$. If the P′ wave precedes the QRS, it does so by no more than 0.12 sec. In cases of digitalis toxicity and junctional tachycardia, there often is AV dissociation.

Causes

Premature junctional complexes, accelerated junctional rhythms, and junctional tachycardia may be caused by the following:
- Ischemia or hypoxia
- Digitalis
- Acute inferior wall MI
- Tricuspid prosthesis
- Rheumatic fever

Clinical implications

In the setting of acute myocardial infarction, a physical assessment may help to define the cause of the junctional premature beats. With bradycardia, AV block, or both, the hemodynamic condition of the patient will dictate the appropriate clinical response. If there is hemodynamic deterioration, the physician should be notified; IV atropine or a pacemaker may be indicated.

If the patient is taking digitalis and has junctional tachycardia, the mortality is approximately 89% if the digitalis is not discontinued.

Rhythm variations

II   PJC

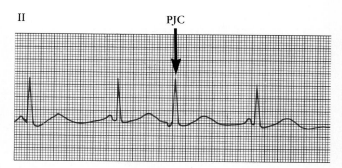

PJC with the P′ preceding the QRS complex

II   PJC

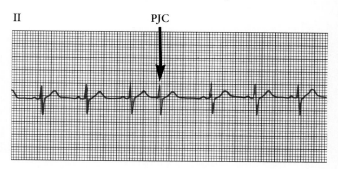

PJC (fourth complex) with the P′ hidden in the QRS
complex; the sinus node is reset with this beat

II   PJC

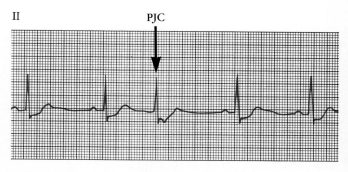

PJC with the P′ following the QRS complex

V₁   P   P

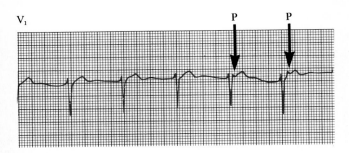

Accelerated idiojunctional rhythm; note that the sinus P
wave is emerging from the end of the QRS in the last two
complexes (the small positive distortion not seen in the first
three QRS complexes)

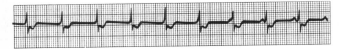

Junctional tachycardia from a suicide attempt with digitalis;
the atrial rate and the junctional rate are similar

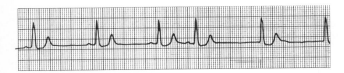

Junctional escape (JE) terminates the pause after the PAC

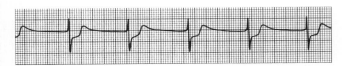

Junctional escape rhythm of 60 beats/min; note the
retrograde P wave in front of the QRS

Treatment

PJCs are not treated. If junctional tachycardia (rate 70-140 beats/min) occurs in a patient taking digoxin, the drug is discontinued, the patient is placed on bed rest (no sympathetic stimulation), and electrolyte replacement may be appropriate.

Acute digitalis overdose (such as suicide attempts) and hemodynamically compromised patients require the digitalis antibody.

Wandering Pacemaker

A wandering pacemaker is an atrial or junctional ectopic rhythm that has approximately the same rate as the sinus node and therefore competes for control of the heart.

Mechanism

The wandering pacemaker may be either a passive escape mechanism or an active intruder; thus the term is merely descriptive and not a primary diagnosis. In association with myocardial infarction, it may occur because of vagotonia.

ECG characteristics

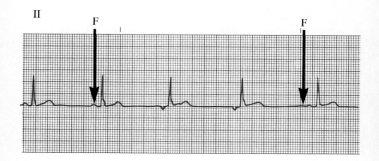

Rate.   Normal or <60 beats/min.

Rhythm.   Slightly irregular.

PR interval.   Normal.

QRS complex.   Normal unless associated with BBB.

Distinguishing features.   A sinus rhythm that gives way to an ectopic atrial or junctional rhythm, often with atrial fusion beats (F) at the transitions; there is retrograde conduction to the atria from the junctional focus.

Causes

- Sinus bradycardia
- Accelerated atrial or junctional rhythm

Clinical implications

If the ectopic rhythm is less than 60 beats/min, it is probably a normal escape mechanism and the only concern is the hemodynamic status of the patient. However, if the ectopic rhythm is more than 60 beats/min, an accelerated ectopic focus is present.

Rhythm variations

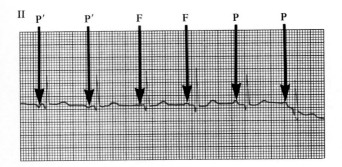

Normal sinus rhythm with an accelerated junctional or atrial rhythm

Treatment

If there is a normal escape mechanism, no treatment is indicated unless there is hemodynamic deterioration, in which case IV atropine may be appropriate.

 ## Atrial Fusion Beats

An atrial fusion beat is a P wave that is a combination of two opposing electrical currents.

Mechanism

Atrial fusion beats result from the presence of two opposing electrical currents (sinus and atrial ectopic) within the same chamber at the same time. The resultant P wave is often narrower and of lesser amplitude than the normal sinus P wave, because opposing currents cancel each other. Atrial fusion is seen in association with atrial parasystole and wandering pacemaker.

ECG characteristics

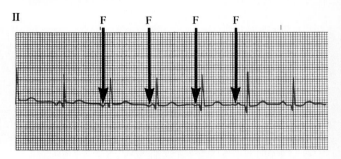

Rate.   That of the underlying rhythm.

Rhythm.   Regular or may be slightly irregular.

PR interval.   The PR interval of the fusion beat is the same as that of the sinus rhythm. The P wave of the fusion beat is sometimes isoelectric or intermediate between the P waves of the fusing impulses.

QRS complex.   That of the underlying rhythm.

Distinguishing features.   There are other atrial ectopic beats in the tracing, and there is reason to believe that one was due at the same time as the sinus P wave.

Causes and clinical implications

- That of the atrial ectopic beat or rhythm.

Rhythm variations

- Atrial parasystole
- Wandering pacemaker

Treatment

Usually none.

Atrial Parasystole

Atrial parasystole is an independent and undisturbable ectopic rhythm whose pacemaker cannot be discharged by impulses of the dominant (usually sinus) rhythm. It is far less common than ventricular parasystole.

Mechanism

Atrial parasystole occurs when an area of enhanced automaticity in the atria is encircled by tissue that is so depressed that the ectopic impulses can exit across it but the sinus impulse cannot enter to discharge it.

ECG characteristics

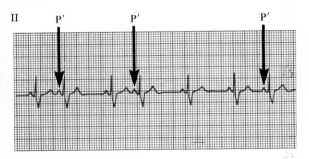

Rate.   That of the underlying rhythm.
Rhythm.   Irregular, because of atrial premature beats.
PR interval.   Normal.
QRS complex.   Normal.
Distinguishing features.   Atrial ectopics with no fixed coupling, interectopic intervals that are multiples of a common denominator, fusion beats.

Cause

■ Myocardial infarction.

 Clinical implications

This is a benign arrhythmia.

Treatment

Usually none.

Paroxysmal Supraventricular Tachycardia (Narrow QRS)

4

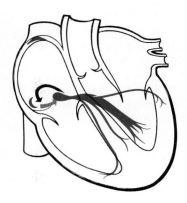

AV nodal reentry tachycardia

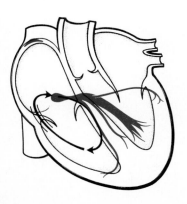

Circus movement tachycardia (AV reciprocating)

Paroxysmal supraventricular tachycardia (PSVT) begins and ends abruptly. It is supported by either an AV nodal reentry circuit (AV nodal reentry tachycardia [AVNRT]) or an AV reentry circuit using the AV node and an accessory pathway (circus movement tachycardia [CMT]). It achieves rates of 170 to 250 beats/min.

It is important to record this tachycardia in multiple leads (at least I, II, III, V_1, and V_6) because of the following:

1. The presence of an accessory pathway is not always manifested with a delta wave during sinus rhythm, in which case the diagnosis can be made only during the tachycardia.
2. During electrophysiological studies (EPS), arrhythmias can be elicited that are not clinically important. It is therefore helpful to know exactly what the clinical arrhythmia is before attempting EPS.
3. The axis of the P' wave during the tachycardia indicates the location of the accessory pathway, providing a guide to the electrophysiologist.
4. An identification of the mechanism of the tachycardia guarantees the symptomatic patient proper referral.

AV Nodal Reentry Tachycardia (AVNRT)
Mechanism

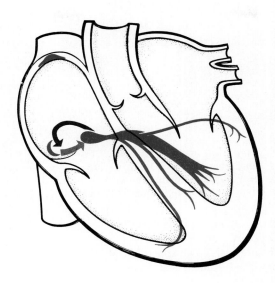

AV nodal reentry is possible because of the existence of two functionally separate pathways approaching the compact node: a slow (posterior) pathway and a fast (anterior) pathway. The refractory period of the slow pathway is the shortest; therefore when an early atrial beat arrives, it may be conducted only down the slow pathway to the ventricles, turning around in the compact AV node to return to the atria via the fast pathway (as shown). The key to ECG recognition of this form of PSVT is understanding that atria and ventricles are activated simultaneously.

Recent studies have demonstrated that the slow pathway is located near the coronary sinus os and along the tricuspid annulus passing into the compact AV node. The fast pathway is located superiorly along the compact node and exits into the atrial septum.

ECG characteristics

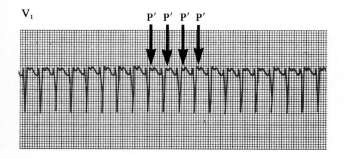

PSVT caused by AV nodal reentry (rate: 250 beats/min)
(Note the P′ wave distorting the end of the QRS, looking
like a tiny r′ — pseudo right bundle branch block [RBBB]
pattern.)

Rate. 170 to 250 beats/min.

Rhythm. PSVT.

PR interval. Not applicable. May be normal in the sinus
rhythm. The P′R interval at the onset of the tachycardia is long
as the impulse uses the slower AV pathway.

QRS complex. Similar to the sinus-conducted QRS
complex; rarely aberrant; often distorted by the P′.

Distinguishing features

1. Prolonged initial P′R interval
2. Narrow QRS
3. P′ waves within the QRS often distorting the end of the
   QRS, looking like terminal s waves in the inferior leads
   and terminal r waves in V_1 (pseudo RBBB pattern)
4. Aberrancy uncommon

Cause

- Usually one early premature atrial complex (PAC)

Clinical implications

AV nodal reentry tachycardia can occur in a normal heart and
is usually a benign mechanism; a small percentage of patients

are, however, refractory to treatment and must be referred to centers skilled at radio-frequency ablation. Patients with PSVT should be instructed in several vagal manuevers.

Bedside diagnosis

- Regular pulse
- "Frog sign" (regular cannon A waves in the jugular venous pulse)
- Constant systolic BP
- Constant intensity of first heart sound
- Carotid sinus massage may terminate PSVT or it may have no effect

Note: The frog sign identifies PSVT but does not differentiate between AVNRT and CMT.

Rhythm variations

Common.   AV nodal reentry using a slow anterograde pathway and a fast retrograde pathway, causing simultaneous atrial and ventricular activation (P' buried within or peeking out at the end of the QRS).

Rare.   AV nodal reentry using a fast anterograde pathway and a slow retrograde pathway, causing atrial activation to follow ventricular activation with a long RP interval (RP > PR). This type of AV nodal reentry should not be confused with the so-called "incessant junctional tachycardia" (p. 140).

Differential diagnosis

See differential diagnosis under Orthodromic Circus Movement Tachycardia.

Emergency treatment*

If *hemodynamically unstable*:

Cardiovert.

Obtain a history.

Record the postconversion 12-lead ECG.

Examine and compare precardioversion and postcardioversion ECG to determine mechanism.

---

*Wellens HJJ, Conover M: The ECG in emergency decision making, Philadelphia, 1992, WB Saunders.

If *hemodynamically stable*:
>   Use vagal stimulation.
>
>   If unsuccessful, give adenosine 6 mg IV rapidly; if unsuccessful, the dosage may be increased to 12 mg and repeated twice 60 seconds apart.
>
>   If unsuccessful, procainamide is used to block either the accessory pathway or the retrograde fast AV nodal pathway.
>
>   If unsuccessful, DC cardioversion is used.

Long-term treatment

When the tachycardia cannot be controlled by vagal maneuvers, the drugs that may be used are digitalis, calcium channel blockers, or beta blockers. Symptomatic patients with AV nodal reentry tachycardia who are resistant to therapy with these drugs are referred for transvenous radio-frequency ablation. Class IA drugs are not used because the risk is higher than with ablation.

 # Orthodromic Circus Movement Tachycardia (CMT) (AV Reciprocating Tachycardia)
Mechanism

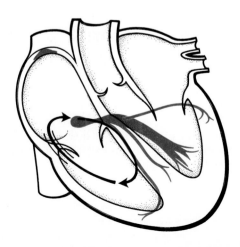

Orthodromic CMT is the second most common cause of PSVT (AVNRT being first) and a common arrhythmia in WPW syndrome. In such patients there are two AV pathways: (1) the normal AV node and His bundle and (2) an accessory pathway. Commonly, a PAC, or less commonly, a premature ventricular beat initiates this tachycardia. The impulse enters the ventricles via the AV node and His bundle (narrow QRS) and returns to the atria via a rapidly conducting accessory pathway, placing the P′ wave close to the preceding QRS. The impulse circulates around and around in this sequence. The most common form uses a rapidly conducting accessory pathway.

ECG characteristics

II

III

V₁

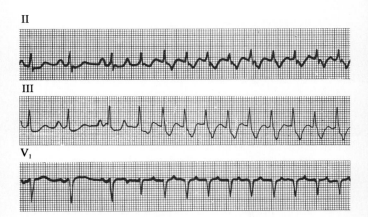

Rate.   150 to 250 beats/min.

Rhythm.   PSVT.

PR interval.   Does not apply because P′ closely follows the R wave, being separate from it. The P′R interval at the outset of the tachycardia is not prolonged as it is in AV nodal reentry tachycardia.

QRS complex.   Normal, unless aberrant.

Distinguishing features

1. Initial P′R interval not prolonged
2. Narrow QRS unless aberrant
3. P′ waves separate from the QRS, but closely follow it

    4. Negative P′ in lead I if left accessory pathway
    5. Aberrancy common
    6. QRS alternans common
    7. Narrow QRS tachycardia that begins and ends abruptly

Causes

- A properly timed initiating PAC or premature ventricular complex (PVC) along with:
- Presence of an accessory pathway

Clinical implications

It is important to make the diagnosis when the patient exhibits CMT, because the 12-lead ECG during sinus rhythm may not show preexcitation (latent or concealed WPW) and because PSVT may result in atrial fibrillation. Patients with symptomatic CMT should be referred to centers skilled in the use of radio-frequency ablation.

Bedside diagnosis

- Regular pulse
- "Frog sign" (regular cannon A waves in the jugular venous pulse)
- Constant systolic BP
- Constant intensity of first heart sound
- Carotid sinus massage may terminate PSVT, or it may have no effect

Note: The frog sign identifies PSVT but does not differentiate between AVNRT and CMT.

Rhythm variations

V_1

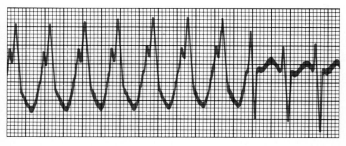

Orthodromic CMT with aberrant ventricular conduction

Differential diagnosis

	AV nodal reentry	CMT
P′ waves	Retrograde; buried in QRS	Separate from QRS; shape depends on accessory pathway location; diagnostic if negative in lead I
Aberrancy	Rare	Common; diagnostic if rate quickens without aberrancy
QRS alternans	Rare	Common

Emergency treatment*

If *hemodynamically unstable*:
>Cardiovert.
>Obtain a history.
>Record the postconversion 12-lead ECG.
>Examine and compare precardioversion and postcardioversion ECG to determine mechanism.

If *hemodynamically stable*:
>Use vagal stimulation.
>If unsuccessful, give adenosine 6 mg IV rapidly; if unsuccessful, the dosage may be increased to 12 mg and repeated twice 60 seconds apart.
>If unsuccessful, procainamide is used to block either the accessory pathway or the retrograde fast AV nodal pathway.
>If unsuccessful, DC cardioversion is used.

Long-term treatment (cure)

Symptomatic patients with CMT are referred for radiofrequency ablation.

*Wellens HJJ, Conover M: The ECG in emergency decision making, Philadelphia, 1992, WB Saunders.

Vagotonic Maneuvers for PSVT

- Gagging.
- Trendelenburg position.
- Valsalva maneuver.
- Squatting. For the young patient, "hunkering down" (squatting with hands gripped across the belly and pulling in) is a fairly easy thing to do and is very effective.
- Carotid sinus stimulation. This maneuver is performed by the physician. The procedure is as follows:
  1. Place the patient in supine position with the neck extended.
  2. Turn the patient's head away from the side to be massaged.
  3. Locate the carotid sinus at the angle of the jaw.
  4. Massage one side at a time, beginning with only slight pressure.
  5. If the patient does not demonstrate hypersensitivity, apply firm pressure with a massaging action for no more than 5 seconds.

  Caution:
  1. Pressure for longer than 5 seconds may be dangerous.
  2. Patients over 65 years of age may respond with long sinus pauses.
  3. Carotid bruits or a history of transient ischemic attacks are contraindications for carotid sinus massage (CSM).
  4. Perform the procedure using ECG monitoring. If an ECG is not available, auscultate the heart during CSM.

Note: (1) Eyeball pressure is ineffective, painful, and dangerous. (2) With time, a vagal maneuver may be ineffective because of the dominance of the sympathetic nervous system.

Effect of Carotid Sinus Massage on Supraventricular Tachycardias*

Type of SVT	Effect of CSM
Sinus tachycardia	Gradual and temporary slowing of sinus rate
Atrial tachycardia	
Paroxysmal	Cessation of tachycardia or no effect
Incessant	Temporary slowing (AV block) or no effect
Atrial flutter	Temporary slowing (AV block)
	Conversion into atrial fibrillation
	No effect
Atrial fibrillation	Temporary slowing (AV block) or no effect
AVNR tachycardia	Cessation of tachycardia or no effect
CMT	Cessation of tachycardia or no effect

*From Wellens HJJ, Brugada P, Bar F: Diagnosis and treatment of the regular tachycardia with a narrow QRS complex. In Kulbertus HE, editor: *Medical management of cardiac arrhythmias,* New York, 1986, Churchill Livingsone.

Ventricular Ectopics

5

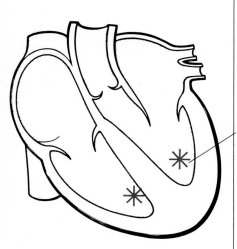

- PVC
- Ventricular tachycardia
- Ventricular fibrillation
- Torsades de pointes
- Accelerated idioventricular rhythm
- Ventricular parasystole
- Ventricular fusion
- Ventricular flutter
- Ventricular escape

Ventricular ectopics take the form of premature ventricular complexes (PVCs), ventricular tachycardia (VT), ventricular fibrillation (VF), accelerated idioventricular rhythm (AIVR), or parasystole.

Treatment

The need for treatment of PVCs or VT depends on the clinical setting, physical symptoms, and arrhythmia pattern, which is evaluated in three major clinical settings: the normal heart, acute ischemic syndromes, and chronic ventricular ectopy.

Therapeutic approaches include the following:

1. No treatment when medically sound.
2. Control of ischemia and heart failure.
3. β-blockers or atropine to modulate sympathetic or parasympathetic tone.
4. Immediate DC cardioversion beginning with synchronized shock of 10 to 50 joules if the VT is associated with hypotension, shock, angina, congestive heart failure, or cerebral hypoperfusion.
5. In hemodynamically stable patients, nonischemic sustained VT is treated with procainamide; ischemic sustained VT is treated with lidocaine. (Use of class I, class III, and some class IV antiarrhythmic agents has a diminishing role.)
6. Implantable devices, antiarrhythmic surgery, radiofrequency ablation (for certain types of VT).
7. Digitalis-induced VT is treated pharmacologically.

Treatment Post-MI

In this clinical setting, PVCs have a low predictive value for life-threatening arrhythmias and there are no data to support treatment of asymptomatic patients with ventricular arrhythmias. In fact, the Cardiac Arrhythmia Suppression Trial (CAST) indicates that mortality is twice as high in the treated population.

The only drug that has been demonstrated to reduce mortality after MI is the β-blocker, which is known to suppress repetitive forms of ventricular ectopy and at times reduce the total frequency of PVCs.

Low-dose amiodarone also may reduce mortality. The side effects of amiodarone are dose related and do not occur if 300 mg or less/day is given.

Intravenous magnesium sulfate or magnesium chloride has been shown to reduce the frequency of clinically important early arrhythmias in patients with MI.

Emergency Response to Broad QRS Tachycardia*

If the patient is *hemodynamically unstable:*

>   Cardiovert.

>   Obtain a history.

>   Examine precardioversion and postcardioversion ECG to determine the etiology and mechanism of the tachycardia.

If the patient is *hemodynamically stable:*

>   Examine the patient for physical signs of AV dissociation.

>   Systematically evaluate the 12-lead ECG.

>   Obtain a history.

If there is *nonischemic ventricular tachycardia:*

>   Give IV procainamide 10 mg/kg body weight IV over 5 min.

If there is *ischemia-related ventricular tachycardia:*

>   Give IV lidocaine 1.5 mg/kg over 3 min.

>>   If this is unsuccessful:

>>>   Cardiovert.

>   Examine precardioversion and postcardioverson ECG to determine etiology of VT.

If there is *supraventricular tachycardia with aberration:*

>   Use vagal stimulation.

>   If this is unsuccessful, administer adenosine 6 mg rapidly IV; if unsuccessful, give 12 mg rapidly (repeat the 12 mg dose once if necessary).

>   If this is unsuccessful, administer procainamide 10 mg/kg body weight IV over 5 min.

>>   If this is unsuccessful:

>>>   Cardiovert.

>   Examine precardioversion and postcardioversion ECG to determine the mechanism.

If *in doubt:*

>   DO NOT give verapamil; give IV procainamide.

If the rhythm is *irregular:*

>   DO NOT give digitalis or verapamil; give IV procainamide.

---

*Wellens HJJ, Conover M: *The ECG in emergency decision making*, Philadelphia, 1992, WB Saunders.

Precordial Thump

Although not recommended by the American Heart Association in unmonitored patients because of the danger of converting VT to VF, in a prospective study in 5000 patients the precordial thump was shown by Caldwell et al. in 1985 to successfully convert 5 cases of VF, 11 cases of VT, 2 cases of asystole, and 2 unknown mechanisms. Conversion from VT to VF was never observed. One or two firm blows are delivered to the sternum at the junction of the middle and lower third. It is not used for unmonitored conscious patients and is immediately abandoned if not successful.

Premature Ventricular Complexes

PVCs are premature ectopic beats originating below the branching of the bundle of His. The focus may be in the ventricular myocardium or in the His-Purkinje system (fascicular PVC).

Mechanism

The mechanism of PVCs may be (1) enhanced normal automaticity within the His-Purkinje system, usually secondary to catecholamines, (2) abnormal automaticity caused by ischemia (with or without infarction), injury, or electrolyte imbalance, (3) reentry as a result of slow conduction, or (4) triggered activity. PVCs also may occur from unknown causes in otherwise healthy hearts.

The full compensatory pause

This measurement implies an uninterrupted sinus rhythm and a nonconducted sinus beat despite the occurrence of a PVC (Figure 5-1). Approximately 50% of the time the sinus rhythm is uninterrupted by the occurrence of a PVC, although the sinus beat immediately following the PVC is usually not conducted and often is not seen because it is buried in the premature complex. A pause is therefore seen after such a PVC. Measuring across the nonconducted sinus P wave, the distance between the conducted P wave preceding the PVC and the one following the PVC is exactly two sinus cycles. This is called a *full compensatory pause*.

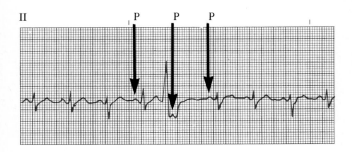

Figure 5-1
PVC with a full compensatory pause. Note that all sinus P waves can be seen.

When the PVC conducts retrogradely to the atria, the pause that follows may be less than "full" (the sinus node being reset by the retrograde P wave) or more than "full" (the sinus node being suppressed by the retrograde P wave) or it may measure exactly "full" because of the timing of the retrograde P wave or the presence or absence of overdrive suppression on the sinus node. Because of all these variables, the full compensatory pause does not prove ventricular ectopy unless the nonconducted sinus P wave can be seen (proving lack of atrial ectopy).

ECG characteristics

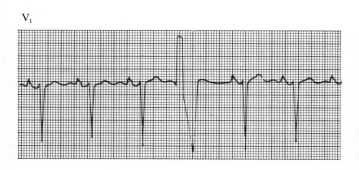

Rate.   That of the underlying rhythm.

Rhythm.   Irregular as a result of the PVC.

PR interval.   That of the underlying rhythm; there is no P wave associated with the PVC.

QRS complex.   That of the PVC is broad (usually >0.12 sec).

Distinguishing features
1. No related P wave
2. Premature, broad QRS complex
3. Large T wave of opposite polarity to the QRS

Causes

- Catecholamines
- Caffeine
- Drugs such as digitalis, epinephrine, isoproterenol, or aminophylline
- Hypokalemia
- Hypomagnesemia
- Hypoxia
- Ischemia
- MI
- Myocardial stretch
- Significant anemia
- Hypotension
- Heart failure
- Bradycardia
- Supraventricular tachycardia

Clinical implications

- In the absence of organic heart disease, PVCs carry little or no cardiovascular risk.
- In acute ischemia, warning PVCs (R on T, multiform, couplets, and more than 30/hr) have a low predictive value for life-threatening forms.
- In chronic ischemic heart disease or cardiomyopathy, PVCs are associated with increased risk of sudden death, especially when the ejection fraction is significantly reduced.

Rhythm variations

II

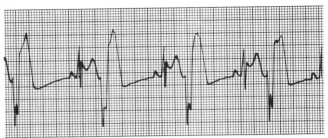

Unifocal PVCs and ventricular bigeminy

V_1

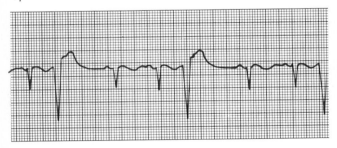

Ventricular trigeminy (two normal and one PVC)

II

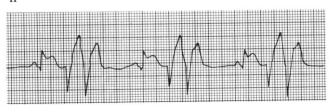

Ventricular trigeminy (one normal and two PVCs)

V₁

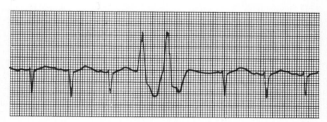

Paired PVCs

II

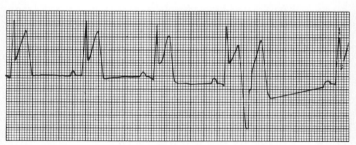

R-on-T phenomenon

II

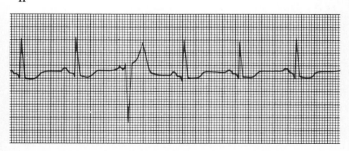

End-diastolic PVC

II

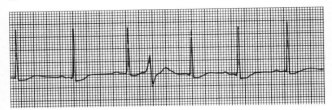

Interpolated PVC

V$_1$

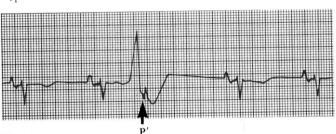

P'

PVC with retrograde conduction to the atria

V$_1$

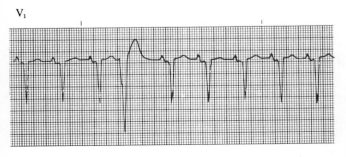

V$_1$-negative PVC

V_1

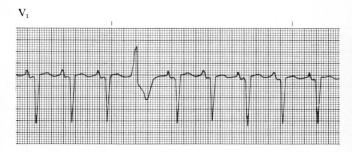

V_1-positive PVC

Differential Diagnosis

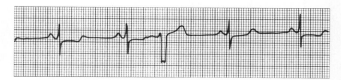

Premature atrial complex (PAC) with aberrant ventricular conduction

Unless a P′ wave can be seen in front of the broad beat (as in this case, distorting the T) or there is morphological proof of ventricular aberrancy, a diagnosis of ventricular ectopy should be made. Note that the compensatory pause is less than full because of premature activation of the atria.

Ventricular Tachycardia

Ventricular tachycardia (VT) is a ventricular rhythm with a rate of 100 to 250 beats/min (some sources state a range of 70 to 250 beats/min, which includes the accelerated idioventricular rhythm). The focus is distal to the branching portion of the bundle of His; hence the QRS is broad.

Mechanism

Reentry, altered automaticity, or triggered activity.

ECG characteristics

V_1

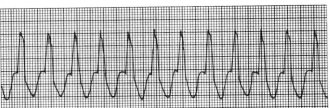

Rate.   100 to 250 beats/min.

Rhythm.   Regular 75% of the time.

PR interval.   Not applicable; approximately 50% of the time atrial activity is independent of ventricular activity (AV dissociation); otherwise there is retrograde conduction to the atria (VA conduction).

QRS complex.   >0.12 sec.

Distinguishing features.   Three or more broad premature ventricular complexes with a T wave of opposite polarity to the main QRS deflection. VT may be monomorphic or polymorphic, vary in a repetitive manner (torsades de pointes), alternate QRS directions (bifascicular VT), be sustained (lasts longer than 30 sec) or nonsustained (lasts less than 30 sec), and may or may not be accompanied by hemodynamic collapse.

Causes (incomplete list)

- Ischemic heart disease
- Congestive and hypertrophic cardiomyopathy
- Primary electrical disease
- Mitral valve prolapse
- Valvular heart disease
- Postoperative coronary artery bypass surgery

- Severe coronary artery disease
- Digitalis, isoproterenol
- May occur in absence of evidence of structural heart disease

Clinical implications

Associated hemodynamic compromise depends on the heart rate, duration, underlying heart disease, and peripheral vascular disease.

Sustained VT usually occurs in patients with reduced ejection fraction, areas of slow intraventricular conduction, left ventricular aneurysm, and previous MI.

Bedside diagnosis

- Regular pulse (in most cases)
- Irregular cannon A waves in the jugular pulse (AV dissociation)
- Regular cannon A waves in the jugular pulse (VA conduction)
- Changing systolic blood pressure
- Changing intensity of first heart sound

Rhythm variations

V₁

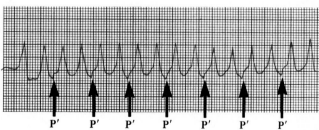

Ventricular tachycardia with retrograde conduction to the atria (2:1)

II

P   P   P   P

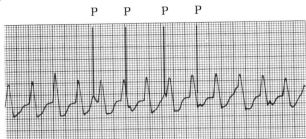

Ventricular tachycardia with AV dissociation (regular, independent P waves during tachycardia are a sign of AV dissociation and support a diagnosis of ventricular tachycardia)

II

F   F

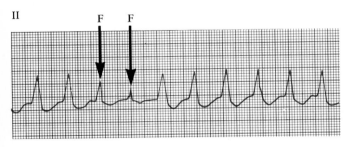

Ventricular tachycardia with ventricular fusion (F)

II

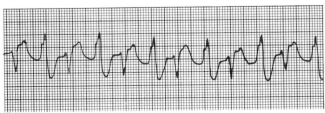

Bifascicular ventricular tachycardia

II

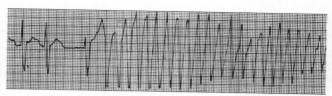

Torsades de pointes (discussed later)

V_1

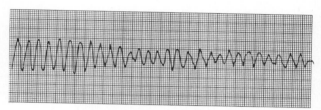

Ventricular flutter/fibrillation

Differential diagnosis

Regular rhythms

1. SVT with preexisting or functional BBB (sinus tachycardia, atrial tachycardia, atrial flutter with fixed AV conduction ratio)
2. PSVT with preexisting or functional BBB (AV nodal reentry tachyardia, circus movement tachycardia using the AV node anterogradely and an accessory pathway retrogradely)
3. SVT with conduction over an accessory pathway (atrial tachycardia, atrial flutter)
4. Antidromic circus movement tachycardia

Irregular rhythms

1. Atrial fibrillation with preexisting or functional BBB
2. Atrial fibrillation with an accessory pathway (p. 143)
3. Atrial flutter with varying AV conduction and preexisting or functional BBB
4. Torsades de pointes (p. 92)
5. Polymorphous VT not associated with a long QT interval

QRS morphology: SVT with aberration vs. VT

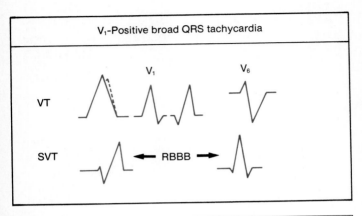

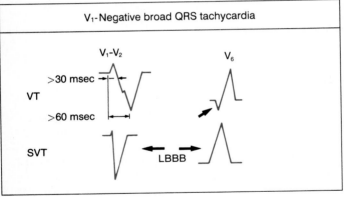

	SVT	VT
Morphology	**In V$_1$-positive:**	**In V$_1$-positive:**
	V$_1$, triphasic (rSR′)	V$_1$ monophasic, biphasic, or "rabbit ear" clue (first peak tallest)
	V$_6$, triphasic (qRS)	V$_6$ R/S ratio <1

	SVT	VT
Morphology	**In V$_1$-negative:**	**In V$_1$-negative:**
	V$_1$ and/or V$_2$: Sharp, narrow r Swift, clean down-stroke	V$_1$ and/or V$_2$: Fat R (>0.03 sec) Slurred S down-stroke S nadir delayed >0.06 sec Any Q in V$_6$
AV dissociation	No	50% of cases
Precordial concordance	Rare	Diagnostic
Fusion or capture beats	No	Supports VT
QRS width	≤ 0.14 sec	>0.14 sec
Heart rate	Not helpful	Not helpful
Axis	Often normal, but may be abnormal	Often abnormal, but may be normal
Hemodynamics	Not helpful	Not helpful
Age	Not helpful	Not helpful

Wide QRS tachycardias that do not follow the morphological rules

- Fascicular VT; often caused by digitalis toxicity, the QRS has an RBBB pattern and a duration of less than 0.14 sec (p. 131).
- VT caused by bundle branch reentry; the QRS has a relatively narrow BBB pattern.
- SVT with AV conduction over an accessory pathway; the QRS is shaped exactly like that of VT; the rhythm is irregular in atrial fibrillation (p. 143).
- Idiopathic VT; two main types have been described. One has an RBBB pattern, a superior axis, and a focus high in the left ventricle; the other has an LBBB pattern, an inferior axis, and a focus in the right ventricular outflow tract.

Ventricular Fibrillation

Ventricular fibrillation is disorganized electrical activity in the ventricles, rendering them incapable of pumping blood.

Mechanism

Individual muscle fibers in the ventricles are depolarizing, but they are disorganized and fail to produce a proper ventricular contraction. The heart quivers and twitches, but does not pump (Figure 5-2).

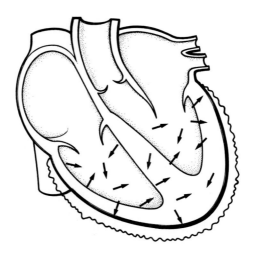

Figure 5-2
Ventricular fibrillation results when there is electrical chaos in the ventricles. It is initiated by a single PVC or is a deterioration of ventricular tachycardia.

ECG characteristics

Rate.   Not applicable.
Rhythm.   Not applicable.
PR interval.   Not applicable.
QRS complex.   Not applicable.

Distinguishing features.   An erratic fibrillatory line without QRS complexes in a patient who becomes faint and loses consciousness, followed by seizures, apnea, and (if untreated) death.

Cause

- Coronary artery disease
- Myocardial ischemia and infarction

Precipitating factors

- VT during ischemia
- Antiarrhythmic drugs
- Hypoxia
- Ischemia
- Atrial fibrillation in patients with accessory pathways
- DC cardioversion
- Improperly grounded equipment in electrically sensitive patients
- Competitive ventricular pacing to terminate VT

Clinical implications

VF is present in 75% of out-of-hospital cardiac arrests, but it has a better prognosis than asystole or bradycardia.

Significant coronary artery disease is present in 75% of resuscitated patients; 20% to 30% develop MI.

Rhythm variations

- Coarse ventricular fibrillation
- Fine ventricular fibrillation

Treatment*

1. Begin cough CPR if patient is awake and able to cough.
2. Defibrillate with 200 joules; repeat once if necessary.
3. If this is successful, administer a bolus of lidocaine 1 mg/kg IV (repeat in 2 min if resuscitation unsuccessful), followed by an infusion of 1 to 4 mg/min.

---

*From Tilkian A, Daily E: *Cardiovascular procedures: diagnostic techniques and therapeutics procedures*, St. Louis, 1986, Mosby–Year Book.

4. If ventricular fibrillation (VF) persists, initiate chest compression and positive-pressure ventilation. Establish IV line.

5. Administer epinephrine 5 to 10 ml of 1:10,000 solution (0.5 to 1 mg) IV or intratracheal.

6. After 30 to 60 sec of ventilation and chest compression, defibrillate with 300 to 400 joules; may repeat once.

7. Administer bretylium 5 mg/kg IV bolus. (Some authorities would begin this sooner.)

8. Administer sodium bicarbonate 1 mEq/kg IV push, especially if metabolic acidosis is documented by arterial blood gases. If VF is terminated within 30 to 60 seconds, significant acidosis does not occur.

9. If VF persists, attempt improvement on ventilation and oxygenation, administer continuous CPR, obtain arterial blood gases, administer further sodium bicarbonate, guided by arterial blood gas results, if available. If not, repeat one-half dose in 10 min.

10. Repeat epinephrine 0.5 to 1 mg IV push.

11. Repeat defibrillation 300 to 400 joules.

12. Consider other drugs — procainamide, magnesium, nitroglycerine, or additional bretylium.

Torsades de Pointes

Torsades de pointes is a VT associated with a prolonged QT interval (usually more than 0.50 sec) that begins with a long-short cycle sequence.

Mechanism

The mechanism is thought to be triggered activity caused by early afterdepolarizations.

ECG characteristics

II

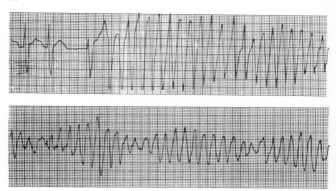

Rate.   200 to 250 beats/min.

Rhythm.   Usually irregular.

PR interval.   Not applicable.

QRS complex.   ≥0.14 sec.

Distinguishing features

1. A VT that has changing amplitudes of the QRS complexes and often begins with a long-short cycle.
2. The QT intervals of the sinus rhythm usually exceed 0.50 sec.
3. There are phasic variations in the electrical polarity of the QRS complex.
4. The tachycardia may be paroxysmal (stopping and then starting up again); the patient may be conscious.

Causes (acquired form)

Anything that lengthens the QT interval, such as the following:

- Antiarrhythmic drugs (quinidine, procainamide, disopyramide, or amiodarone, sotalol, N-acetylprocainamide)
- Hypokalemia
- Hypomagnesemia
- Liquid protein diet and starvation
- Profound bradycardia
- Central nervous system pathology
- Unilateral alteration of sympathetic tone
- Phenothiazines or tricyclic antidepressants
- Cardiac ganglionitis
- Mitral valve prolapse

Clinical implications

Preventive care (acquired form):

- Measure the QT interval on admission to the CCU.
- If the patient is on quinidine, procainamide, disopyramide, or amiodarone, alert all personnel to the importance of QT measurements.
- If possible, secure a QT measurement from a previous ECG.
- Notify the physician if the QT lengthens more than 33% or beyond 0.50 sec (uncorrected).
- If torsades de pointes develops, prepare for pacing, IV magnesium sulfate, or magnesium chloride.

The congenital form may or may not be associated with sensorineural deafness.

Differential diagnosis

Because of the therapeutic implications, it is very important to distinguish between a VT with morphology similar to that of torsades de pointes but that occurs without QT prolongation and is often ischemia related.

Treatment

1. IV magnesium sulfate or magnesium chloride (IV push: 2 g over 1 to 2 min; IV infusion: 1 to 2 g/hr for 4 to 6 hr)
2. Temporary overdrive ventricular or atrial pacing

Accelerated Idioventricular Rhythm

The accelerated idioventricular rhythm (AIVR) is an ectopic ventricular rhythm with a rate of 40 to 100 beats/min.

Mechanism

The arrhythmia often is seen in the setting of acute myocardial infarction and is thought to be benign unless it is the result of digitalis toxicity. The mechanism is altered automaticity.

ECG characteristics

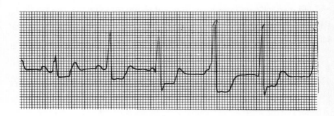

Rate.   60 to 110 beats/min.

Rhythm.   Regular or irregular.

PR interval.   Not applicable, but that of the underlying rhythm may be normal or shortened because of fusion beats.

QRS complex.   > 0.12 sec.

Distinguishing features.   A ventricular ectopic rhythm that begins gradually (nonparoxysmal), often with fusion beats because the rate is similar to that of the sinus node.

Cause

- Reperfusion (spontaneous or after thrombolysis) phase of myocardial infarction.

Clinical implications

AIVR is a reperfusion arrhythmia (spontaneous or because of thrombolysis) occurring at the moment of reperfusion of a previously occluded coronary artery; it is seen also in the setting of digitalis toxicity.

It is transient, intermittent, lasts less than a minute, and does not appear to impact the clinical course unless AV dissociation results in hemodynamic impairment.

Rhythm variations

The configuration of the ventricular ectopic varies according to the location of reperfusion. For example, multiple QRS configurations implies reperfusion of the left anterior descending coronary artery (the QRS may be relatively narrow); a V_1-negative configuration excludes circumflex occlusion; and an electrical axis between 0 and 180 degrees virtually rules out a right coronary artery occlusion.

Treatment

None, unless the patient is symptomatic or there is a more serious concurrent arrhythmia.

 # Ventricular Fusion Complexes

A ventricular fusion complex results when two impulses collide within the ventricles.

Mechanism

Ventricular fusion beats result from the presence of two opposing electrical currents (sinus and ventricular ectopic) within the same chamber at the same time. The resulting ECG complex often is narrower and of lesser amplitude than the ectopic beat alone. Ventricular fusion often is seen in association with ventricular parasystole, accelerated idioventricular rhythms, and end-diastolic PVCs.

ECG characteristics

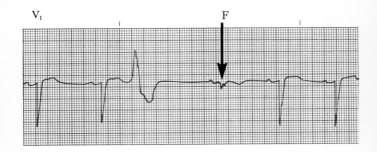

Rate. That of the underlying rhythm.

Rhythm. Regular.

PR interval. PR interval of the fusion beat may be the same as or shorter than that of the sinus rhythm, but it is never more than 0.06 sec shorter than the dominant PR interval.

QRS complex. Normal in the underlying rhythm, but may be anything in the fusion beats.

Distinguishing features. Other ventricular ectopic beats in the tracing and reason to believe that one was due at that moment.

QRS of the fusion beat has a contour intermediate between that of the fusing impulses.

Cause

■ That of the ventricular ectopic beat or rhythm.

Clinical implications

In the setting of acute myocardial infarction, occasional ventricular fusion beats (end-diastolic PVCs) may warn of congestive heart failure. It is at this point in the cardiac cycle that the stretching of myocardial tissue is the greatest.

Generally, ventricular fusion beats have the nursing implications of the ventricular ectopic beat or rhythm itself.

Rhythm variations

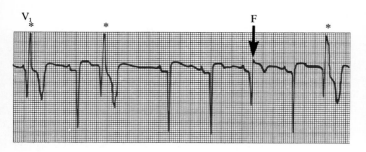

Ventricular parasystole

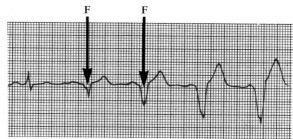

Accelerated idioventricular rhythm

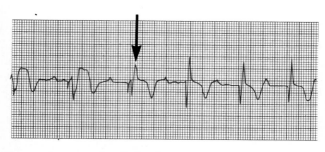

Electronic pacemaker fusion beat

II

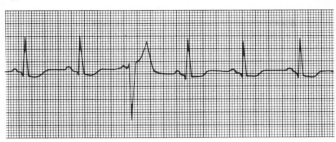

End-diastolic PVCs

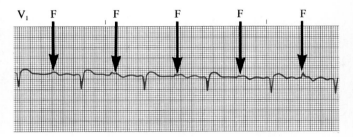

Bigeminal end-diastolic PVCs

Treatment

Usually none.

Ventricular Parasystole

Ventricular parasystole is an independent and undisturbable ectopic rhythm whose pacemaker cannot be discharged by impulses of the dominant (usually sinus) rhythm.

Mechanism

Parasystolic rhythms develop because of an area of abnormal automaticity surrounded by an area of depressed tissue, which blocks any incoming impulse and keeps the pacemaker from being extraneously discharged. This protected ectopic pacemaker fires at regular intervals and captures the ventricles whenever they are nonrefractory; otherwise the ectopic focus goes undetected on the surface ECG (Figure 5-3). The parasystolic focus is not totally unresponsive to the electrical influence surrounding it and may be affected so that its rhythm is not precisely regular.

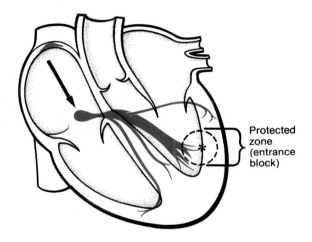

Protected zone (entrance block)

Figure 5-3
In ventricular parasystole there is a protected ectopic focus in the ventricles that keeps its own rate and is not discharged by extraneous impulses, although it may be electrogenically influenced by them.

ECG characteristics

V₁

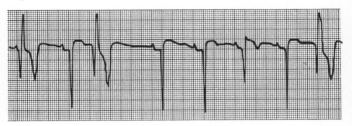

Rate.   That of the underlying rhythm.
Rhythm.   Irregular, as a result of the extrasystoles.
PR interval.   Normal in the underlying rhythm.
QRS complex.   Normal in the underlying rhythm; broad in the parasystolic beats.
Distinguishing features.   Interectopic intervals that have a common denominator, fusion beats, no fixed coupling.

Clinical implications

Because this is a benign arrhythmia, observe the patient for complications, but no treatment is indicated.

Even though it seems likely that a parasystolic beat will eventually activate the ventricles during the T wave, actually when a parasystolic impulse coincides with the T wave, it seldom becomes a manifest beat.

Rhythm variations

- Fixed coupling in parasystole if the rates of the two pacemakers happen to be mathematically related
- No fixed coupling, but interectopic intervals are not exact multiples, because the ectopic focus is influenced, but not reset, by the sinus impulses

Differential diagnosis

Accelerated idioventricular rhythm.

Treatment

Usually none.

Ventricular Flutter

Ventricular flutter is a very rapid ventricular tachycardia without a clearly formed QRS complex.

Mechanism

This arrhythmia is a deterioration of ventricular tachycardia, representing severe disorganization within the ventricles.

ECG characteristics

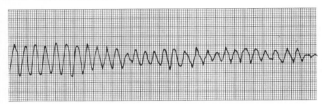

Rate.   150 to 300 beats/min (average about 200 beats/min).

Rhythm.   Regular.

PR interval.   Not applicable.

QRS complex.   Not applicable.

Distinguishing features.   A zig-zag configuration instead of clearly defined QRS complexes.

Causes

- Myocardial infarction
- Myocardial ischemia

 Clinical implications

An interim arrhythmia between ventricular tachycardia and fibrillation; hemodynamic collapse is present.

This arrhythmia has the same clinical and nursing implications as ventricular fibrillation.

Treatment

Same as for ventricular fibrillation.

 Ventricular Escape

Ventricular escape is characterized by an ectopic beat that originates in the ventricles and follows a long pause.

Mechanism

The ventricular escape beat is not abnormal in itself, but the fact that it is necessary is abnormal. Such a beat implies that (1) the sinus node or AV conduction failed and (2) the junctional escape mechanism failed. A junctional escape beat is next in line after the sinus node for pacing function.

ECG characteristics

II

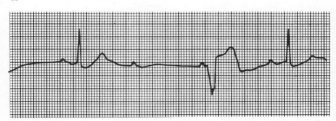

> **Rate.**   That of the underlying rhythm.
> **Rhythm.**   Irregular.
> **PR interval.**   Not applicable to this beat.
> **QRS complex.**   >0.12 sec (the escape beat).
> **Distinguishing feature.**   A broad QRS that follows a
long pause.

Cause

- Failure of the sinus node or AV conduction along with failure of the junctional escape mechanism.

Clinical implications

The ventricular escape beat is a good thing in itself. Attention must be directed at (1) why there was not a normal sinus-conducted beat and (2) why there was not a junctional escape beat instead of the ventricular escape.

Differential diagnosis

Late junctional escape with phase 4 aberration.

Treatment

That of the underlying problem.

Aberrant Ventricular Conduction

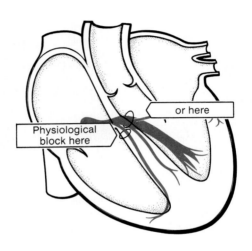

Physiological block here

or here

 Aberrant Ventricular Conduction

Aberrant ventricular conduction is a transient bundle branch block, hemiblock, or both, which is commonly though not exclusively caused by an abrupt shortening of cycle length (phase 3 aberration). It also may be caused by a lengthening of the cycle (phase 4 aberration) and may be sustained by retrograde concealed conduction.

Mechanism

In aberrant ventricular conduction, one of the main bundle branches or one of the fascicles is blocked. Commonly this transient block occurs in the right bundle branch but also may take the form of hemiblock or LBBB.

Clinical implications

It is critically important to differentiate between aberrancy and ectopy because of the following:

- Verapamil mistakenly given to a patient in ventricular tachycardia (VT) may cause death or at least seriously compromise the patient.
- Mistaking SVT for VT leaves the patient who has an accessory pathway without a diagnosis and without referral for a cure with radio-frequency ablation.

Rhythm variations

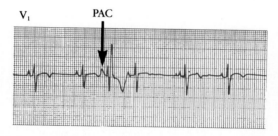

PAC with RBBB aberrancy

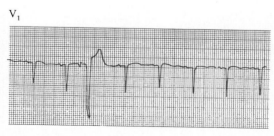

PAC with LBBB aberrancy

V₁

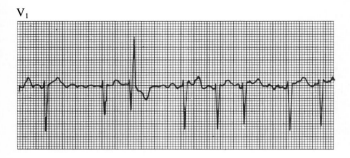

Atrial fibrillation with RBBB aberrancy

II

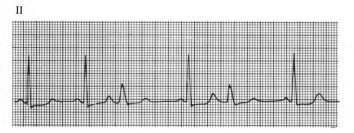

Bigeminal PACS with aberrancy

V₁

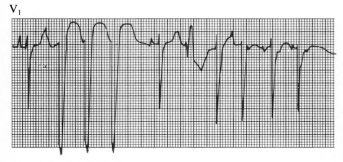

RBBB and LBBB aberrancy

V₁

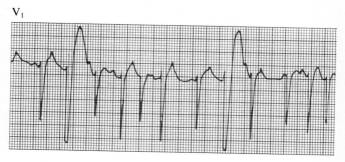

Chaotic atrial tachycardia with LBBB aberrancy

Differential Diagnosis

V₁

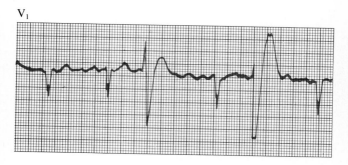

Atrial fibrillation with ventricular ectopics (When the broad complexes in V_1 are negative, an R wave broader than 0.03 sec indicates ventricular ectopy [third complex]).

V₁

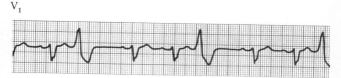

Sinus rhythm with PVCs. (When the broad complexes in V_1 are positive, a monophasic R wave indicates ventricular ectopy.)

Treatment

Aberrant ventricular conduction is not treated. Treatment of ventricular tachycardia is dictated by the clinical setting (see pp. 75-77). PSVT is recorded, terminated, and the mechanism is determined (see pp. 67 and 71). Long-term treatment for symptomatic PSVT may involve radio-frequency ablation.

AV Block

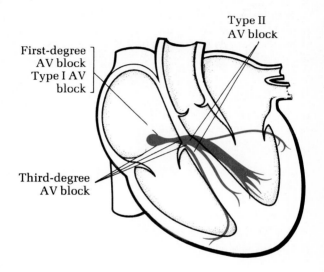

First-degree AV block / Type I AV block

Type II AV block

Third-degree AV block

Atrioventricular (AV) block is present when the atrial impulses are not conducted to the ventricles or are conducted with delay when the possibility for conduction exists. It is divided into first, second, and third degree. AV block commonly is located in the AV node, bundle of His, or bundle branches.

Determination of the Site of AV Block

The level of AV block can be determined noninvasively by using atropine, exercise or catecholamines, or carotid sinus massage.

AV nodal block. Atropine and exercise or catecholamines improve AV conduction, and carotid sinus massage worsens it.

Subnodal block. Atropine and exercise or catecholamines worsen AV conduction, and carotid sinus massage improves it.

Treatment

Temporary or permanent pacemaker insertion is indicated in patients with symptomatic bradyarrhythmias.

For short-term therapy, atropine helps if the lesion is AV nodal. Catecholamines (e.g., isoproterenol) may improve conduction, but as a general rule they are not used for patients with acute MI.

 First-Degree AV Block

First-degree AV block is prolonged AV conduction with all P waves being conducted and all PR intervals the same.

Mechanisms

- Prolonged PR, normal QRS = conduction delay in the AV node.
- Prolonged PR, BBB pattern = AV nodal and/or His-Purkinje pathology.
- Occasionally the conduction delay is within the atria.

ECG characteristics

II

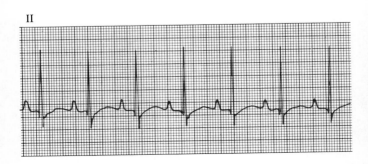

Rate. Normal.

Rhythm. Regular.

PR interval. > 0.20 sec.

QRS complex. Normal (unless there is another block in the bundle branches).

Distinguishing features. Prolonged PR; all beats conducted.

Causes

- Digitalis
- Ischemic heart disease
- Inferior wall MI
- Hyperkalemia
- Acute rheumatic fever
- A normal variant

Clinical implications

If the first-degree AV block is in the setting of acute inferior wall MI, it is usually transient.

Bedside diagnosis

- Long a-c wave interval in the jugular venous pulse
- Diminished intensity of the first heart sound
- PR shortens with atropine, exercise, or catecholamines if AV nodal
- PR lengthens with carotid sinus massage if AV nodal
- PR lengthens with atropine, exercise, or catecholamines if subnodal
- PR shortens with carotid sinus massage if subnodal

Second-Degree AV Block

In second-degree AV block, not all atrial impulses are conducted to the ventricles. There are two types of second-degree AV block: type I (Mobitz I) and type II (Mobitz II).

Type I

In type I AV block there is incremental conduction delay at the level of the AV node until a P wave is not conducted (also called *AV Wenckebach* or *Mobitz I*).

Mechanism

Type I AV block with a normal QRS is a function of the AV node.

ECG characteristics

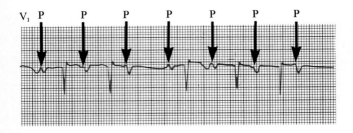

Rate.   Normal.

Rhythm.   Irregular.

PR interval.   Lengthens until a beat is dropped. The first PR of the series is usually >0.20 sec.

QRS complex.   Normal.

Distinguishing features.   Lengthening PR intervals, shortening RR intervals, and pauses that are less than twice the shortest cycle. There is group beating.

Causes

- Digitalis
- Ischemic heart disease
- Inferior wall myocardial infarction
- Increased vagal tone, as in athletes

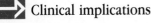 Clinical implications

Type I AV block is usually associated with acute inferior wall MI; it is usually transient and does not require a pacemaker. In this setting, a high-grade block indicates more damage and a higher mortality.

Bedside diagnosis

- A widening a-c interval in the jugular venous pulse terminated by a pause, and an *a* wave not followed by a *v* wave

- Gradually diminishing intensity of the first heart sound
- Improved conduction with atropine, exercise, or catecholamines

Rhythm variations

II

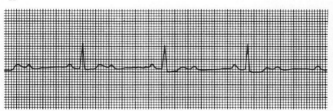

2:1 block is neither type I nor type II; it may be nodal or subnodal (If it is AV nodal, conduction improves with exercise, atropine, or catecholamines; if it is subnodal, it improves with carotid sinus massage.)

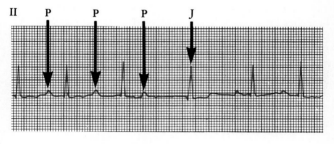

Wenckebach with junctional escape

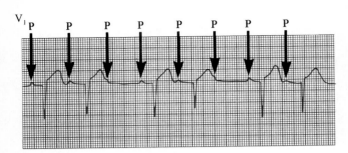

3:2 Wenckebach

Differential diagnosis

Concealed junctional extrasystoles can mimic second-degree AV block.

Type II

Type II AV block is conduction delay at the level of the bundle branches.

Mechanism

There is a delay in AV conduction at the level of the bundle branches; therefore the QRS is usually broad. The PR is normal as long as conduction at the level of the AV node is not compromised as well.

ECG characteristics

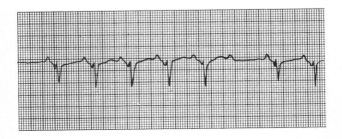

Rate. Normal.
Rhythm. Irregular.
PR interval. Normal; some P waves are not conducted.
QRS complex. Broad.
Distinguishing features. Fixed, normal PR intervals, broad QRS complexes, and dropped beats.

Causes

- Severe conduction system disease
- Anterior wall myocardial infarction

Clinical implications

The physician should be notified, because type II AV block may be an indication for a pacemaker.

Type II AV block often precedes syncope and complete AV block.

Type II AV block is usually associated with acute anterior wall MI, may require temporary or permanent pacing, and carries with it a high mortality.

Bedside diagnosis

- Intermittent pauses in the heartbeat
- In the jugular venous pulse some *a* waves are not followed by *v* waves
- Constant first heart sound

Rhythm variations

II

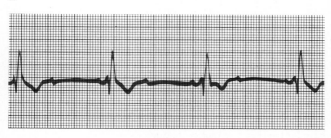

2:1 AV conduction with a broad QRS and short PR

Differential diagnosis

Concealed junctional extrasystoles can mimic second-degree AV block.

 ## Third-Degree (Complete) AV Block

Third-degree, or complete, AV block occurs when the atrial impulse is unable to pass into the ventricles.

Mechanism

There is pathology at the AV node, bundle of His, or bundle branches such that atrial impulses cannot pass. Thus the atria and the ventricles beat independently of each other (one form of AV dissociation). The atrial focus may be sinus or ectopic; the ventricular focus is located below the pathology (His bundle or below).

ECG characteristics

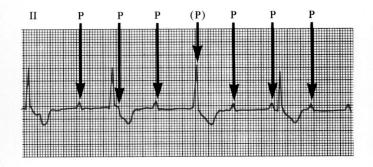

Rate.   < 40 beats/min in acquired complete block; faster in congenital complete block.

Rhythm.   Usually regular, but may vary.

PR interval.   Not applicable.

QRS complex.   Narrow or broad, depending on the location of the escape pacemaker and the condition of the interventricular conduction system.

Distinguishing features.   Regular QRS complexes at a rate of 40 to 60 beats/min and AV dissociation.

Causes

- Chronic degenerative conduction disease
- Digitalis toxicity
- Myocardial infarction

Clinical implications

If the block is secondary to inferior wall myocardial infarction, the escape pacemaker is a dependable junctional one with a rate of about 40 to 60 beats/min. This is usually a reversible condition, and a pacemaker may not be needed.

If the block is in the setting of acute anteroseptal myocardial infarction, the condition is usually more serious.

In either case, the physician should be notified.

Rhythm variations

V₁

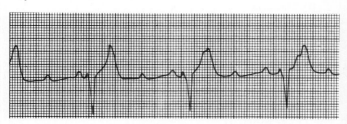

Third-degree AV block with an idioventricular rhythm

V₁

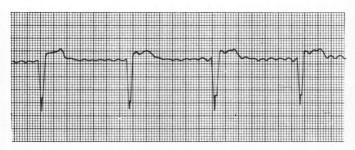

Atrial fibrillation with third-degree AV block

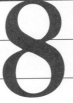
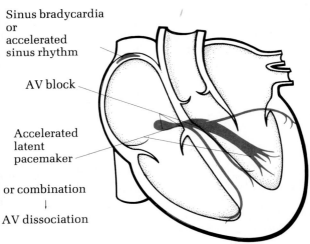

Sinus bradycardia
or
accelerated
sinus rhythm

AV block

Accelerated
latent
pacemaker

or combination
↓
AV dissociation

 ## AV Dissociation

Atrioventricular (AV) dissociation is the independent beating of atria and ventricles. It is important to remember that the term *AV dissociation* is not a diagnosis. The primary disorder is indicated by the ECG diagnosis, which may be either clinically insignificant, such as sinus bradycardia and junctional escape in an athlete, or clinically significant, such as an accelerated idiojunctional rhythm or complete AV block. Thus the cause must always be identified.

Mechanism

AV dissociation is the result of a basic disturbance in impulse formation, conduction, or both. In any case, the atria beat independent of the ventricles in any type of supraventricular rhythm.

ECG characteristics

Rate.   That of the ventricular pacemaker.

Rhythm.   Usually regular but may be irregular if there is occasional conduction (capture).

PR interval.   Not applicable.

QRS duration.   Narrow or broad, depending on the ventricular pacemaker.

Distinguishing features.   Independently beating atria and ventricles. In some cases the P waves may appear to "walk into" R waves.

Causes

- Sinus bradycardia
- Acceleration of a subsidiary pacemaker
- AV block
- Any combination of the above

Clinical implications

Because the causes vary from normal conditions to abnormal ones, it is important to determine the mechanism and cause.

If the QRS complexes are narrow, the ventricular pacemaker is junctional (bundle of His). Determine the rate to determine if this represents a normal escape mechanism or an accelerated focus.

If the QRS complexes are broad, the ventricular pacemaker is ventricular below the branching of the bundle of His; or it may be junctional with bundle branch block.

If there is an accelerated idiojunctional focus, digitalis may be the cause and the physician should be notified. Electrolyte and digitalis levels may be ordered, although "therapeutic" digitalis blood levels do not necessarily indicate absence of toxicity.

Bedside diagnosis

- Varying intensity first heart sound
- Irregular cannon *a* waves in the jugular venous pulse
- Beat-to-beat varying systolic pressure

Rhythm variations

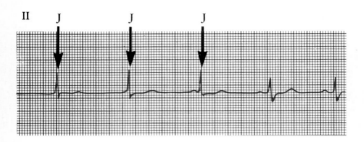

Sinus bradycardia with a junctional escape rhythm

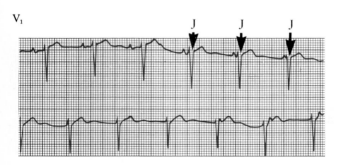

Accelerated idiojunctional rhythm

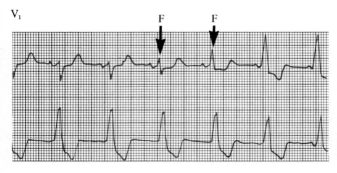

Accelerated idioventricular rhythm (F = fusion)

II

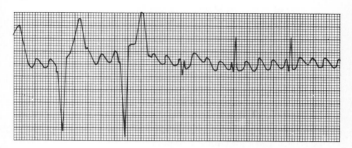

Atrial flutter with an accelerated idioventricular rhythm
(The last three are capture beats, the first of which is a
fusion beat.)

II

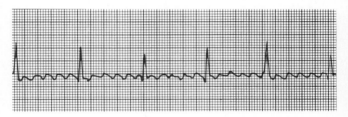

Atrial flutter with AV dissociation and two capture beats
(first and fifth)

II

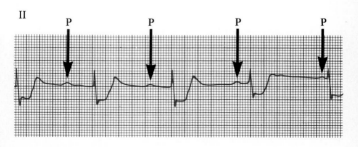

Complete AV block

V₁

C

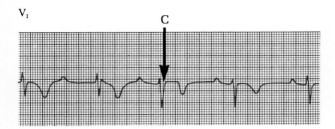

High-grade second-degree AV block with an idiojunctional pacemaker and one capture beat

Differential diagnosis

See "Rhythm variations."

Treatment

If the AV dissociation is a result of an accelerated subsidiary pacemaker, a clinical assessment is indicated and the cause is treated.

If there is sinus bradycardia with a junctional escape focus, no treatment may be indicated as long as there is no hemodynamic deterioration.

Digitalis Dysrhythmias

9

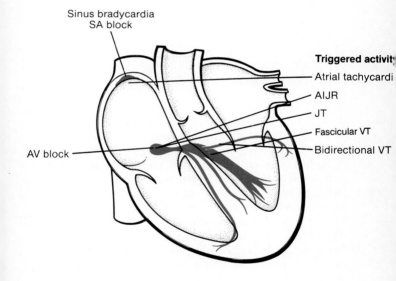

Sinus bradycardia
SA block

Triggered activity

Atrial tachycardia

AIJR

JT

Fascicular VT

Bidirectional VT

AV block

Digitalis is used as an antiarrhythmic because it lengthens the refractory period of the AV node, slowing the ventricular response to atrial fibrillation and atrial flutter. Associated arrhythmias are sinus bradycardia, SA block, AV block, atrial tachycardia, junctional tachycardia, and fascicular VT.

Mechanism

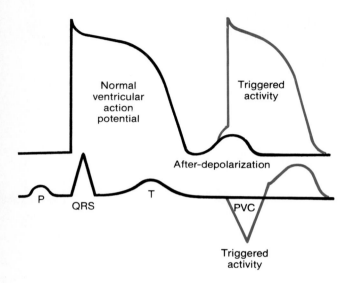

1. Digitalis causes an accumulation of sodium within the cardiac cell by inhibiting the Na^+-K^+ ATPase pump.
2. The high concentration of intracellular Na^+ causes an increase in intracellular Ca^{++} by altering the function of the Na^+-Ca^{++} exchange, as well as Ca^{++} release from the sarcoplasmic reticulum and other intracellular stores.
3. This increase in intracellular Ca^{++} triggers a transient inward Na^+ current, which causes an oscillation at the end of phase 3 of the action potential (delayed afterdepolarization).
4. If this oscillation, called a *delayed afterdepolarization*, reaches threshold potential for the fast sodium channels, tachycardias result. Such a mechanism is called *triggered activity* to differentiate it from ectopic rhythms caused by automaticity.
5. Catecholamines induce an increase in intracellular Ca^{++} and thus potentiate the occurrence of tachycardias.

ECG recognition

Be alert for the following four features:
1. Bradycardia when previously normal or fast (caused by SA or AV block)
2. Tachycardia when previously normal (causes: atrial tachycardia, AV junctional tachycardia, fascicular VT)
3. Unexpected regularity when irregularity is expected (caused by complete AV block with a regular AV junctional rhythm in a patient with atrial fibrillation or atrial flutter)
4. Regular irregularity, such as the group beating of ventricular bigeminy, SA or AV Wenckebach, or combinations of these

Systematic evaluation

1. Ask the patient about dosage, other medications, and symptoms.
2. Seek information from the family about patient's symptoms.
3. If there are P waves, monitor in lead II, evaluating for atrial tachycardia and/or AV dissociation. The P waves of atrial tachycardia will be upright in this lead.
4. If there is AV dissociation, look at lead V_1 to see if there is a junctional or a fascicular rhythm.
5. If there is atrial fibrillation, monitor in lead V_1 for junctional rhythm vs. fascicular VT.
6. If there is atrial flutter, evaluate lead II or V_1 for signs of AV dissociation; if present, look at V_1 for junctional rhythm vs. fascicular VT.

Physical signs of digitalis toxicity (partial list)

- Noticeable changes in color vision (especially red/green) and print when reading (change in clearness)
- Sleeping problems
- Changes in behavior, such as lack of energy or memory lapses (pseudodementia)

Clinical implications

The emergencies created by digitalis frequently are not apparent, especially since "therapeutic" blood levels do not guarantee nontoxicity. Diagnosis and correct management are critical because of the high mortality associated with unrecognized or poorly managed cases of digitalis toxicity (100% in atrial and in ventricular tachycardia [VT]; 70% in junctional tachycardia). The arrhythmias of digitalis toxicity are the result of (1) block in conduction (both in the sinoatrial [SA] and atrioventricular [AV] junctional regions) and (2) delayed afterdepolarizations that, when achieving threshold potential, result in triggered activity (atrial, AV junctional, and fascicular tachycardia).

Conditions that may promote digitalis dysrhythmias

- Increased sympathetic tone
- Hypokalemia
- Hypercalcemia
- Hypomagnesemia
- Diuretics
- Ischemia and reperfusion
- Increased wall tension
- Heart failure

Treatment*

1. Discontinue the drug.
2. Correct potassium and magnesium deficits.
3. Prescribe bedrest (no sympathetic stimulation).
4. Begin continuous ECG monitoring.
5. Do not use carotid sinus massage (may result in VF).
6. Phenytoin and a pacemaker or digitalis antibodies may be used, especially if the patient is hemodynamically unstable.
7. Ventricular pacing is indicated in symptomatic bradycardia and during treatment with phenytoin because suppression of the tachycardia may be followed by asystole.

AVOID beta-stimulation (stress, anxiety, exercise, sympathomimetic drugs), atropine, carotid sinus massage, and fast or sudden cessation of pacing.

*Wellens HJJ, Conover M: The ECG in emergency decision making, Philadelphia, 1992, WB Saunders.

Common Digitalis Dysrhythmias
Atrial Tachycardia with Block

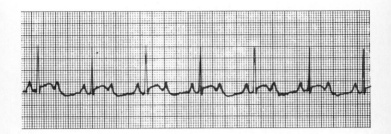

Rate.   130 to 250 beats/min (atrial); the ventricular rate depends on the AV conduction ratio.

Rhythm.   May be irregular.

PR interval.   Often prolonged because of the digitalis effect on AV conduction.

QRS complex.   Narrow, unless there is an associated BBB or fascicular VT.

Distinguishing features
1. 2 : 1 AV block or AV Wenckebach
2. P axis is superior to inferior (P' upright in lead II)
3. Ventriculophasic PP intervals
4. Nonparoxysmal

Rhythm variations

- Double tachycardias: atrial tachycardia and junctional tachycardia; atrial tachycardia and fascicular VT
- Atrial tachycardia with 1 : 1 conduction or varying degrees of AV block

Differential diagnosis

	Atrial tachycardia	AVNRT	CMT	Sinus tachycardia
P waves	In digitalis toxicity; like sinus Ps	Retrograde; buried in QRS; may distort the QRS	Follows the QRS; shape depends on accessory pathway location	In front of QRS
Rhythm	Nonparoxysmal; may be irregular in digitalis toxicity	Paroxysmal; regular	Paroxysmal; regular	Gradual acceleration
Rate (beats/min)	130-250	170-250	170-250	>100; but >90 may also be abnormal

AVNRT, AV nodal reentry tachycardia; *CMT*, circus movement tachycardia.

Junctional Tachycardia

Junctional tachycardia is an ectopic SV rhythm with a rate of 70 to 140 beats/min (it may manifest itself at a slower rate depending on the rate of the sinus node). When the rate is <100 beats/min, it is sometimes called *accelerated idiojunctional rhythm.*

Mechanism

In digitalis toxicity the focus of this arrhythmia is at the distal AV node where the bundle of His begins. There is usually AV block caused by the effect of digitalis.

ECG characteristics

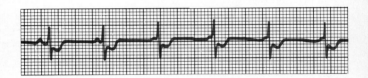

Rate.   70 to 140 beats/min.
Rhythm.   Usually regular.
PR interval.   Not applicable.
QRS complex.   Narrow.
Distinguishing features
1. Nonparoxysmal
2. Rate increase with exercise
3. Nodoventricular block or no effect from carotid sinus massage
4. AV dissociation (usually)
5. Gradual onset
6. Rate rarely exceeds 140 beats/min

Rhythm variations

II

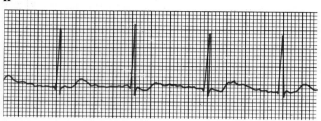

Atrial fibrillation with junctional tachycardia (accelerated idiojunctional rhythm)

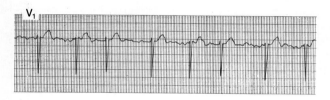

Atrial fibrillation with junctional tachycardia and Wenckebach exit block (group beating)

V₁

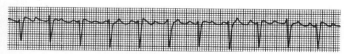

Atrial flutter with junctional tachycardia; note the changing flutter-R relationship (a sign of AV dissociation in atrial flutter)

Fascicular VT

Fascicular VT is common to digitalis toxicity. The focus of this arrhythmia is in one of the fascicles of the bundle branches, usually in the anterior or posterior division of the left bundle branch.

Mechanism

Because the focus is located in the proximal specialized conduction system, the resulting QRS is not as broad as in other types of VT. The shape of the QRS is that of RBBB with axis deviation when the impulse begins in one of the fascicles of the left bundle branch.

ECG characteristics

V_1

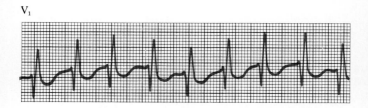

Rate. 90 to 160 beats/min.
Rhythm. Usually regular.
PR interval. Not applicable.
QRS complex. 0.12 to 0.14 sec; RBBB.
Distinguishing features
1. RBBB shape
2. QRS: 0.12 to 0.14 sec
3. Axis deviation (right or left)

Rhythm variations

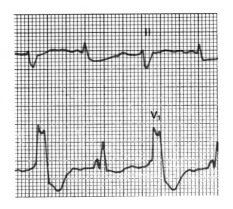

Bifascicular VT (There is an RBBB pattern in lead V_1 and alternating right and left axis deviation.)

Sinus Bradycardia and SA Block

V_1

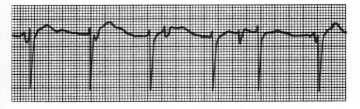

Sinus bradycardia with an AIJR (There is one capture beat [the 5th complex].)

The sinus bradycardia may be profound and associated with AV block, junctional tachycardia, or fascicular VT.

V_2

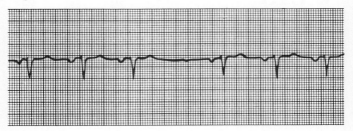

SA Wenckebach

SA block is diagnosed because there are dropped P waves. In SA Wenckebach there is group beating of the P waves and the PP intervals become shorter before the dropped P wave.

AV Wenckebach

II

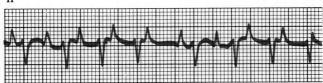

Atrial tachycardia with AV Wenckebach (Note the lengthening P'R intervals and the dropped beat.)

AV Wenckebach conduction is a typical feature of digitalis toxicity and may be associated with atrial tachycardia. In its classical form it is recognized because of group beating, lengthening PR intervals, shortening RR intervals, and a pause that is less than twice the shortest cycle

Wolff-Parkinson-White Syndrome

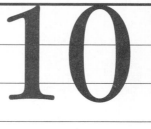

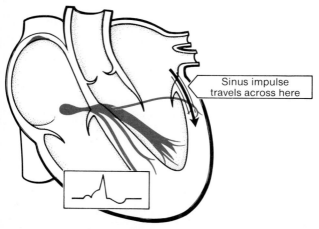

10

Sinus impulse travels across here

Wolff-Parkinson-White (WPW) is a group of ECG findings (short PR, delta wave, and broad QRS) associated with a tendency to develop PSVT, which may deteriorate into atrial fibrillation or flutter with conduction down the accessory pathway and heart rates as high as 200 to 300 beats/min. When the ECG findings exist without the associated tachycardia, the term *WPW pattern* is used. Mahaim fibers are discussed also.

 Accessory Pathways

Patients with WPW syndrome have one or more extra muscle connections between an atrium and a ventricle (accessory pathway), which may result in an *overt* WPW pattern or may be *latent* or *concealed*.

In *overt WPW syndrome,* there is preexcitation of the ventricles because of an accessory pathway connecting the atria and the ventricles, with conduction possible in both directions across it. This permits the sinus impulse to enter the ventricles without AV delay and outside the conduction system, producing a typical ECG.

When the accessory pathway is *latent*, the ECG is normal during sinus rhythm because the impulse arrives in the ventricles faster via the AV node than by the accessory pathway.

When the accessory pathway is *concealed*, the ECG during sinus rhythm is normal because impulses can be conducted only retrogradely over the accessory pathway.

Thus in overt, latent, and concealed WPW syndrome, AV reciprocating tachycardia (circus movement tachycardia) is possible using the AV node anterogradely and the accessory pathway retrogradely. However, during atrial fibrillation the patient with concealed WPW syndrome is protected from life-threatening ventricular rates because anterograde accessory pathway conduction does not take place.

ECG characteristics

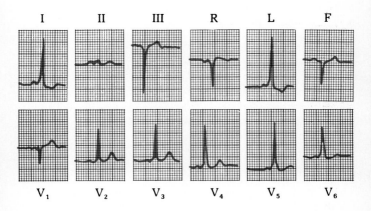

Overt WPW syndrome

Rate.   Normal.

Rhythm.   Regular.

PR interval.   < 0.12 sec.

QRS complex.   > 0.11 sec.

Distinguishing features.   Short PR, broad QRS, delta wave (slurred beginning to the QRS), and a tendency to PSVT and atrial fibrillation or flutter. There may be secondary T wave changes.

Latent and concealed accessory pathways

Rate.   Normal.

Rhythm.   Regular.

PR interval.   Normal.

QRS complex.   Normal.

Distinguishing features

1. *Latent:* Normal PR, normal QRS, and a tendency to PSVT; if atrial fibrillation or flutter develops, AV conduction proceeds anterogradely across the accessory pathway, resulting in a rapid, broad QRS tachycardia.
2. *Concealed:* Normal PR, normal QRS, and a tendency to PSVT; if atrial fibrillation or flutter develops, AV conduction is normal (down the AV node) and the QRS narrow because there is anterograde block in the accessory pathway.

Cause

- Congenital

 ## Clinical implications

Symptomatic patients should be referred to a center skilled in the use of radio-frequency ablation. This technique offers a complete cure.

Arrhythmias Common to WPW Syndrome

The most common arrhythmias in WPW syndrome are orthodromic circus movement tachycardia (CMT) using a rapidly conducting accessory pathway and atrial fibrillation. Less common are atrial flutter, antidromic CMT, and orthodromic CMT using a slowly conducting accessory pathway.

Orthodromic CMT (Rapidly Conducting Accessory Pathway)
Mechanism

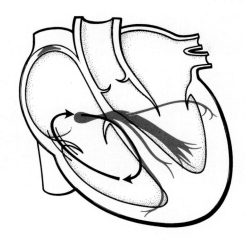

Note that there are two AV pathways: (1) the normal AV node and His bundle and (2) an accessory pathway. Commonly, a PAC or, less commonly, a PVC initiates this tachycardia. The impulse enters the ventricles via the AV node and His bundle (narrow QRS) and returns to the atria via a rapidly conducting accessory pathway, placing the P′ wave close to the preceding QRS. The impulse circulates around and around in this sequence. The most common form uses a rapidly conducting accessory pathway; a less common form uses a slowly conducting accessory pathway. Both forms have a typical ECG.

ECG characteristics (rapidly conducting accessory pathway)

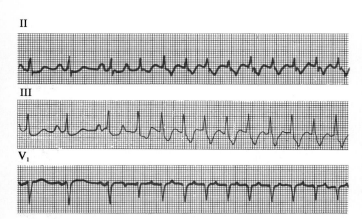

Rate.   150 to 250 beats/min.

Rhythm.   PSVT.

PR interval.   Does not apply because P′ closely follows the R wave, being separate from it. The P′R interval at the outset of the tachycardia is not prolonged as it is in AV nodal reentry tachycardia.

QRS complex.   Normal, unless aberrant.

Distinguishing features

1. Initial P′R interval not prolonged
2. Narrow QRS unless aberrant
3. P′ wave separate from the QRS but closely follows it
4. Negative P′ in lead I if left-lateral accessory pathway
5. Aberrancy common
6. QRS alternans common
7. Narrow QRS tachycardia that begins and ends abruptly

Causes

- A properly timed initiating PAC or PVC and
- Presence of an accessory pathway

Clinical implications

It is important to make the diagnosis when the patient exhibits CMT because the 12-lead ECG during sinus rhythm may not show preexcitation (latent or concealed WPW) and because PSVT may result in atrial fibrillation. Patients with symptomatic CMT should be referred to centers skilled in the use of radio-frequency ablation.

An ECG record of PSVT in at least five leads is very important, not only to make the differential diagnosis, but also because at the time of electrophysiological studies, clinically irrelevant arrhythmias can be elicited. However, if the PSVT has already been recorded, much information can be gleaned, many unknowns eliminated, and procedure time shortened.

Bedside diagnosis

- Regular pulse
- "Frog sign" (regular cannon A waves in the jugular venous pulse)
- Constant systolic BP
- Constant intensity of first heart sound
- Carotid sinus massage may terminate PSVT or it may have no effect

Note: The frog sign identifies PSVT but does not differentiate between AVNRT and CMT.

Rhythm variations

V_1

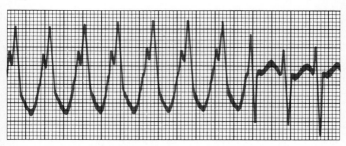

Orthodromic CMT with aberrant ventricular conduction

Differential diagnosis

The differential diagnosis between CMT and AV nodal reentry tachycardia is discussed in Chapter 4.

Emergency treatment*

1. If *hemodynamically unstable*:
     Cardiovert.
     Obtain a history.
     Record the postconversion 12-lead ECG.
     Examine and compare precardioversion and postcardioversion ECG to determine mechanism.
2. If *hemodynamically stable*:
     Use vagal stimulation.
     If unsuccessful, give adenosine 6 mg IV rapidly; if unsuccessful, the dosage may be increased to 12 mg and repeated twice 60 seconds apart.
     If unsuccessful, procainamide is used to block either the accessory pathway or the retrograde fast AV nodal pathway.
     If unsuccessful, DC cardioversion is used.

Long-term treatment (cure)

Symptomatic patients with CMT are referred for radio-frequency ablation.

 ## Orthodromic CMT (Slowly Conducting Accessory Pathway)
ECG characteristics

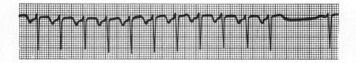

    Rate.   > 150 beats/min.
    Rhythm.   Described as "incessant;" "persistent;" "permanent."
    PR interval.   RP' greater than P'R.

*Wellens HJJ, Conover M: *The ECG in emergency decision making*, Philadelphia, 1992, WB Saunders.

QRS complex.   Normal.

Distinguishing features.   Patient is in the tachycardia 90% of the time; the RP' is longer than the P'R; often causes congestive heart failure.

Clinical implications

Although this form of orthodromic CMT is very rare, it is extremely important to recognize it, because a complete cure is available for this debilitating arrhythmia.

Treatment (cure)

Radio-frequency ablation of the slowly conducting accessory pathway, which is usually located posterior septally.

Antidromic CMT

Antidromic CMT is a rare form of PSVT.

Mechanism

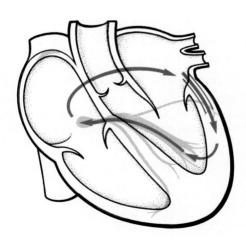

The reentry circuit uses the accessory pathway anterogradely and the bundle of His and AV node retrogradely, producing a tachycardia identical in appearance to VT.

ECG characteristics

Rate.   >170 beats/min.
Rhythm.   Regular.
QRS complex.   Identical to VT.
Distinguishing features.   Broad QRS tachycardia identical in form to VT.

Causes

- A critically timed PAC or PVC
- Presence of an accessory pathway

 ## Clinical implications

Patients with antidromic CMT often have multiple accessory pathways and should be referred to centers skilled in the use of radio-frequency ablation techniques.

Differential diagnosis

Must be differentiated from VT by electrophysiological studies.

Emergency and long-term treatment

1. Same as for orthodromic CMT
2. Radio-frequency ablation

 ## Atrial Fibrillation with Preexcitation

Atrial fibrillation is a common arrhythmia in patients with WPW syndrome. It results in a rapid, irregular, broad QRS tachycardia that may deteriorate into ventricular fibrillation.

Mechanism

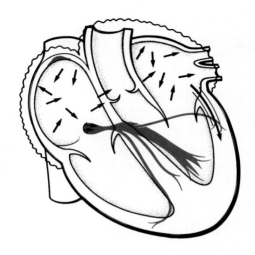

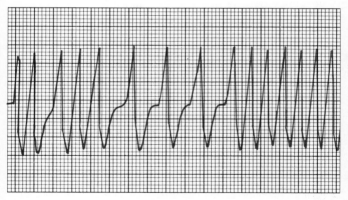

The frequent and erratic atrial impulses of atrial fibrillation are conducted into the ventricles over the accessory pathway. The ventricular rate is over 200 beats/min, being determined by the refractory period of the accessory pathway, which varies among individuals.

ECG characteristics

Rate.   > 200 beats/min.
Rhythm.   Irregular.
QRS complex.   Identical to VT.
Distinguishing features.   Fast, Broad, Irregular (FBI); identical to VT except that it is irregular.

Causes

- PSVT or without warning
- Presence of an accessory pathway

 Clinical implications

This is a life-threatening arrhythmia. These patients are referred to a center skilled in the technique of radio-frequency ablation.

Differential diagnosis

Differentiated from VT because of the irregularity, rate, and history.

Emergency treatment*

1. *If hemodynamically unstable*: DC cardioversion.
2. *If hemodynamically stable*: Administer procainamide IV 10 mg/kg body weight over 5 min (if the rate does not slow, DC cardioversion).

Danger: Do not use digitalis or calcium channel blockers (they may accelerate the ventricular rate).

Long-term treatment (cure)

Radio-frequency ablation.

 PSVT Resulting from Mahaim Fibers

Mahaim fibers are anomalous tracts between the AV node or bundle of His and the ventricles.

---

*Wellens HJJ, Conover M: *The ECG in emergency decision making*, Philadelphia, 1992, WB Saunders.

Mechanism

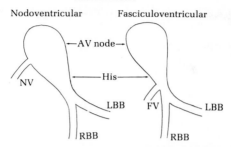

Mahaim fibers

	Nodoventricular	Fasciculoventricular
Site of origin:	AV node	**His bundle or bundle branches**
PR:	Short or normal	**Normal (isolated FV)**
QRS:	Anomalous—fusion	**Anomalous—fixed**

From Gallagher JJ et al: Role of Mahaim fibers in cardiac arrhythmias in man, *Circulation* 64:176, 1981. By permission of the American Heart Association, Inc.

Historically, two main anatomic types of Mahaim fibers are described: nodoventricular (NV) arise from the AV node, whereas fasciculoventricular (FV) arise from the bundle of His or the bundle branches. The NV connection does not support PSVT.

Recent information suggests a right atrioventricular accessory pathway with AV nodal-like conducting properties. PSVT results from a circuit pathway using the accessory pathway anterogradely and the AV node retrogradely.

ECG characteristics

Rate. Normal.

Rhythm. Regular.

PR interval. Short or normal (nodoventricular connection); normal (fasciculoventricular connection).

QRS complex. Fusion beat; varies in morphology (nodoventricular connection); anomalous (fasciculoventricular connection).

Cause

- Congenital anomalous AV connections

Clinical implications

The arrhythmias seen in this condition may deteriorate into ventricular fibrillation.

Emergency treatment

Same as for PSVT.

Wellens Syndrome

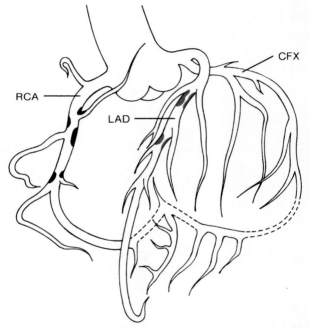

11

Wellens Syndrome

Wellens syndrome is a group of five signs that permit ECG recognition of critical proximal LAD stenosis:

- Unstable angina
- Little or no enzyme elevation
- No pathological precordial Q waves
- Little or no ST segment elevation in V_2 and V_3
- ST segment in V_2 and V_3 turns down into a progressively deep, symmetrical, inverted T

Note: ECG signs are seen during painfree intervals.

ECG recognition

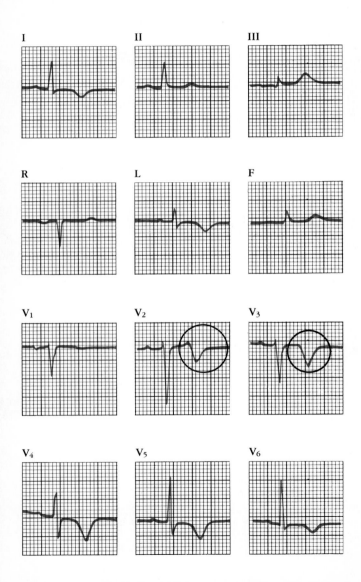

Clinical implications

Because of the life-preserving interventions now available, such as bypass graft and coronary angioplasty, early aggressive treatment of patients with critical proximal stenosis of the left anterior descending (LAD) coronary artery or severe main-stem and three-vessel disease is most desirable.

Management

Emergency arteriography is indicated; the patient may be a candidate for emergency percutaneous transvenous coronary angioplasty (PTCA) or for coronary artery bypass graft.

ECG Recognition of Left Mainstem and Three-Vessel Disease

I
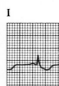

II
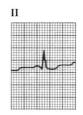

III
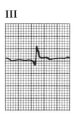

R
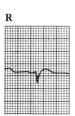

L
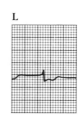

F
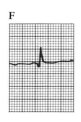

V₁
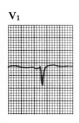

V₂
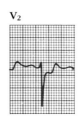

V₃
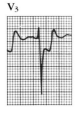

V₄
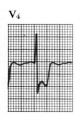

V₅
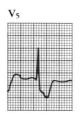

V₆
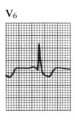

Left mainstem and three-vessel coronary artery disease can be diagnosed in patients with the following:

- Unstable angina
- ST elevation in aV_R and V_1
- ST depression in eight or more leads

Note: In 32% of patients, these ECG signs are seen only during pain.

Management

Emergency arteriography is indicated; the patient may be a candidate for emergency percutaneous transvenous coronary angioplasty (PTCA) or for coronary artery bypass graft.

Bundle Branch Block and Hemiblock

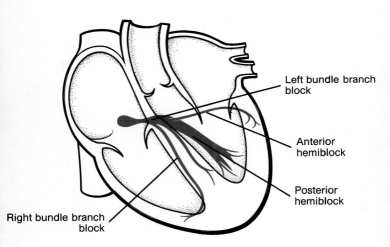

12

Left bundle branch block

Anterior hemiblock

Posterior hemiblock

Right bundle branch block

A block at the level of the bundle branches (right or left bundle branch block [RBBB or LBBB]) causes the ventricles to be activated in sequence instead of simultaneously. This produces a broad QRS complex that has a typical diagnostic morphology in V_1 and V_6. The left bundle branch is divided into two main fascicles (anterior and posterior); a block of one is called *hemiblock*.

Anatomy and Physiology

In normal intraventricular activation, both ventricles are activated at the same time, producing a narrow QRS. The bundle branches speed the impulse to the ventricles. Therefore when a bundle branch is blocked, the ventricle it serves is activated late and the QRS is 0.12 sec or more. Hemiblock is a block of one division (anterior or posterior) of the left bundle branch.

Right Bundle Branch Block
Pathophysiology and mechanism

The right bundle branch is much smaller than the left and can be compromised by a lesser lesion; thus RBBB frequently is clinically benign. When the right bundle branch is blocked, septal and left ventricular activation are normal but the impulse arrives under V_1 later than it should, causing the R wave to be late (late intrinsicoid deflection) in that lead (Figure 12-1).

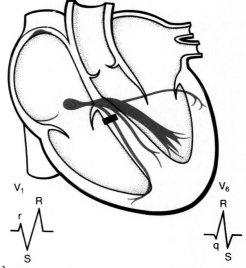

Figure 12-1
In RBBB, activation of both ventricles in sequence causes a broad complex with a late R wave in V_1 and an S wave in V_6.

ECG characteristics

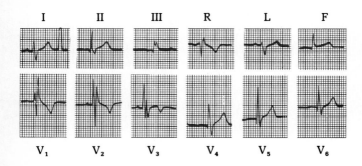

I	II	III	R	L	F
V₁	V₂	V₃	V₄	V₅	V₆

Rate. Normal.

Rhythm. Normal.

PR interval. Normal.

QRS complex. 0.12 sec or greater; classical pattern in V_1 is rSR′.

Distinguishing features. A broad QRS that is mainly positive in V_1 and has an intrinsicoid deflection of 0.07 sec or later in that lead. In I, aV_L, and V_6, the only abnormality is a broad S wave. There are secondary T wave changes.

Causes

- Found in otherwise normal hearts
- Lenegre's disease
- Lev's disease
- Ischemic heart disease
- Chagas' disease
- Rheumatic disease
- Syphilis
- Trauma
- Tumors
- Cardiomyopathy
- Cogenital lesions
- Surgical correction of tetralogy of Fallot or ventricular septal defect
- Acute heart failure
- Acute myocardial infarction
- Acute coronary insufficiency

- Acute infection
- Right heart catheterization
- Intracardiac catheter in position

Clinical implications

In the setting of acute anteroseptal myocardial infarction, such a diagnosis is associated with a mortality of 65% and often the anterior division of the left bundle is compromised also. When bundle branch block develops in this clinical setting, efforts toward reperfusion are very aggressive.

If the RBBB is in the setting of apparent health, there is no adverse effect.

An RBBB pattern (rSR′ in V_1) is also seen when the right ventricle is activated late (fascicular VT and idiopathic VT); when a P′ wave distorts the end of the QRS (AV nodal reentry tachycardia); and when there is a functional block of the right bundle branch (e.g., SVT with RBBB aberration).

Pattern variations

V_1

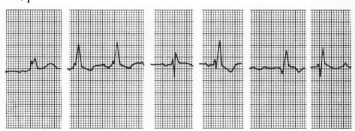

Different shapes of RBBB in V_1

V_1

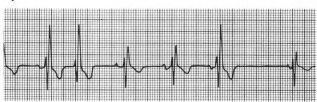

Incomplete RBBB has the QRS shape but not the duration

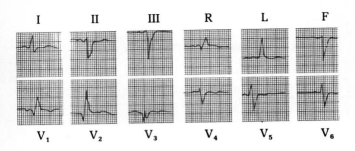

RBBB and anteroseptal myocardial infarction; anterior hemiblock is present also

V₁

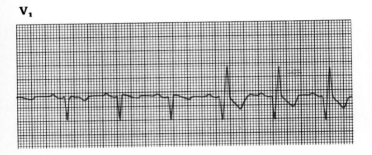

When the rate increases from 80 to 82 beats/min (the "critical rate"), rate-related RBBB results

Treatment

None, although in the setting of acute anteroseptal myocardial infarction, a pacemaker may be indicated.

 Left Bundle Branch Block
Pathophysiology and mechanism

LBBB (Figure 12-2) usually reflects serious underlying heart disease because a large lesion is required to block the left bundle branch. This bundle is thick and broad and has a blood supply from two sources: the right and the left coronary arteries. Typically the lesion is in the common left bundle before it branches.

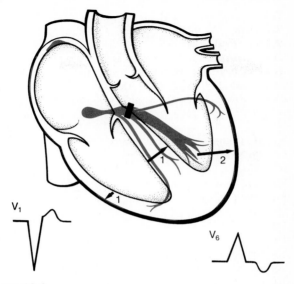

Figure 12-2
In LBBB, activation of both ventricles in sequence causes a very broad complex that is negative in V_1 and positive in V_6.

When the left bundle branch is blocked, both initial and terminal forces are abnormal. The septum is activated from right to left; the left ventricle is activated from the currents in the right ventricle.

ECG characteristics

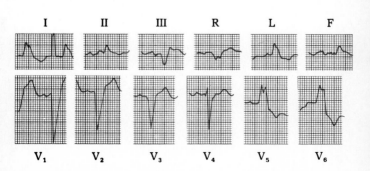

Rate.   Normal.

Rhythm.   Normal.

PR interval.   Normal.

QRS complex.   0.12 sec or greater.

Distinguishing features.   A broad QRS that is mainly negative in V_1. In I, aV_L, and V_6, there is an R wave, no q wave, and no S wave. There are secondary T wave changes.

Causes

- Found in otherwise normal hearts
- Lenegre's disease
- Lev's disease
- Ischemic heart disease
- Rheumatic disease
- Syphilis
- Trauma
- Tumors
- Cardiomyopathy
- Congenital lesions
- Severe aortic stenosis
- Acute heart failure
- Acute myocardial infarction
- Acute coronary insufficiency
- Acute infection

Clinical implications

The physician should be notified if LBBB develops in the setting of acute anteroseptal myocardial infarction.

The prognosis depends on the underlying cause.

Pattern variations

V₁

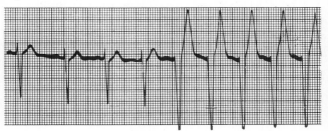

When the rate increases to 100 beats/min (the "critical rate"), rate-related LBBB results

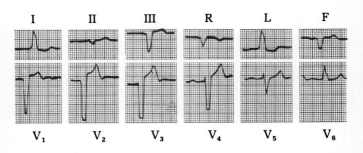

LBBB with left axis deviation occurs in about 30% of cases of LBBB and is thought to indicate more extensive damage to the anterior fascicle of the left bundle

Differential diagnosis

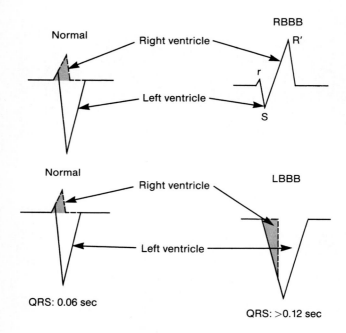

Normal conduction, right bundle branch block, and left bundle branch block are compared above in lead V_1. The dotted lines indicate hidden events on the ECG. For example, right ventricular activation is normally effaced by left ventricular activation.

Treatment

None, although in the setting of acute anteroseptal myocardial infarction, a pacemaker may be indicated.

Anterior Hemiblock

Anterior hemiblock is a block of the anterior superior division of the left bundle branch.

Pathophysiology and mechanism

Anterior hemiblock (Figure 12-3) is more common and less serious than posterior hemiblock. The anterior fascicle of the LBB is long and thin, and has only one blood supply, as does the RBB, and is in the outflow tract of the left ventricle, whereas the posterior fascicle is broad, has two blood supplies, and is not subjected to the mechanical stresses of the anterior division.

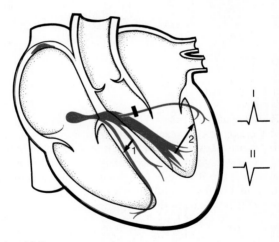

Figure 12-3
Left anterior hemiblock (LAH) causes left axis deviation.

When the anterior fascicle is blocked, the impulse activates the ventricles via the posterior inferior fascicle; this produces left axis deviation.

ECG characteristics

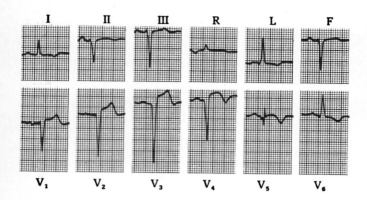

Rate.   Normal.
Rhythm.   Normal.
PR interval.   Normal.
QRS complex.   Normal (lengthens by only 0.02 sec).
Distinguishing features.   Left axis deviation of more than −45 degrees (generally accepted); a terminal R wave in aV_R and aV_L; the R wave in aV_R is later than the R in aV_L; a q wave in I and aV_L and an r wave in II, III, and aV_F; increased QRS voltage in the limb leads.

Causes

- Found in otherwise normal hearts
- Lenegre's disease
- Lev's disease
- Aortic valve calcification
- Cardiomyopathy
- Ischemic heart disease
- Acute myocardial infarction
- Cardiac catheterization
- Selective coronary arteriography
- Hyperkalemia
- Surgical correction of tetralogy of Fallot

Clinical implications

The physician should be notified if anterior hemiblock develops in the setting of acute anteroseptal myocardial infarction.

The prognosis depends on the underlying cause.

Pattern variations

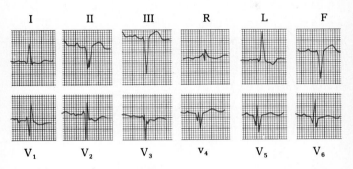

RBBB and anterior hemiblock

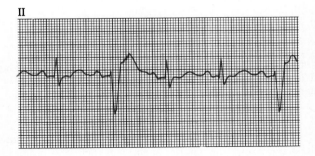

Intermittent anterior hemiblock with first-degree AV block and RBBB

Treatment

Usually none, although in the setting of acute anteroseptal myocardial infarction, a pacemaker may be indicated.

Posterior Hemiblock

Posterior hemiblock is a block of the posterior inferior division of the left bundle branch.

Pathophysiology and mechanism

Posterior hemiblock (Figure 12-4) has more serious clinical implications because it implies the compromise of two blood supplies (right and left coronary arteries) and damage to a broad inferior conduction system in the left ventricle.

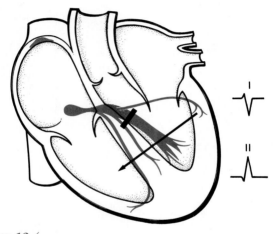

Figure 12-4
Left posterior hemiblock (LPH) has right axis deviation and is less common than LAH because the posterior fascicle has two blood supplies and the anterior only one.

When the posterior fascicle is blocked, the impulse gets into the ventricles via the anterior superior fascicle; this produces right axis deviation.

ECG characteristics

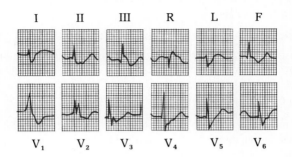

I   II   III   R   L   F

V_1 V_2 V_3 V_4 V_5 V_6

Rate.   Normal, but may be accelerated or slow as a result of another conduction.

Rhythm.   Normal.

PR interval.   Normal.

QRS complex.   Normal (lengthens by only 0.02 sec).

Distinguishing features.   Right axis deviation of more than + 120 degrees, a q wave in II, III, and aV_F, an r wave in I and aV_L, increased QRS voltage in the limb leads.

Causes

- Lenegre's disease
- Lev's disease
- Aortic valve calcification
- Cardiomyopathy
- Ischemic heart disease
- Acute myocardial infarction
- Cardiac catheterization
- Selective coronary arteriography
- Hyperkalemia

Clinical implications

The physician should be notified if posterior hemiblock develops in the setting of acute anteroseptal myocardial infarction, in which case it is associated with RBBB and a poor prognosis. Complete subnodal AV block develops in 90% of cases.

Usually posterior hemiblock is accompanied by RBBB, which may be intermittent.

Treatment

In the setting of acute anteroseptal myocardial infarction, a pacemaker may be indicated.

 Trifascicular Block

Trifascicular block is a complete or incomplete pathological conduction impairment located simultaneously in the three main fascicles of the intraventricular conductive systgem—the right bundle branch and the anterior and posterior divisions of the left bundle branch (Figure 12-5).

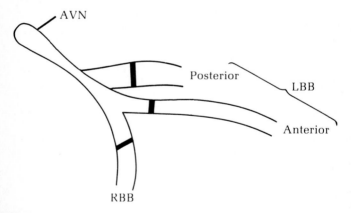

Figure 12-5
Trifascicular block. When this type of block is complete in all fascicles, third-degree AV block results.

Pathophysiology and mechanism

A pathological condition in three of the fascicles of the intraventricular conduction system is ominous and implies compromise of two coronary arteries: the anterior descending left and the posterior descending right. The anterior descending left coronary artery supplies the RBB, the anterior division of the LBB, and part of the posterior division of the LBB, the remainder of which is supplied by the posterior descending right coronary artery.

If the block is complete across all fascicles (there are actually four), the escape pacemaker will be below that level and therefore will be a slow ventricular pacemaker whose rate is incompatible with life. If the block is not complete, the supraventricular impulses arrive in the ventricles either with first-degree AV block or type II second-degree AV block.

ECG characteristics

Rate.   That of the underlying rhythm; if there is complete block, the ventricular rate is < 40/min.

Rhythm.   That of the underlying rhythm.

PR interval.   That of the underlying rhythm.

QRS complex.   Broad.

Distinguishing features.   This condition may take many forms:

1. Complete AV block
2. RBBB + left anterior hemiblock (LAH) + first- or second-degree AV block
3. RBBB + left posterior hemiblock (LPH) + first- or second-degree AV block
4. LBBB + first- or second-degree AV block
5. Various combinations of these

Causes

- Coronary artery disease
- Lenegre's disease
- Lev's disease

Clinical implications

If the trifascicular block is complete, the patient suddenly experiences profound bradycardia and emergency pacemaker insertion is indicated.

If the trifascicular block is incomplete (see "Distinguishing Features"), notify the physician and prepare for elective pacemaker insertion.

Pattern variations

- Complete AV block with a slow idioventricular rhythm
- RBBB + LAH + first-degree or type II second-degree AV block
- RBBB + LPH + first-degree or type II second-degree AV block
- LBBB + first-degree or type II second-degree AV block
- Various combinations of these

Treatment

A pacemaker may be inserted.

Myocardial Infarction

13

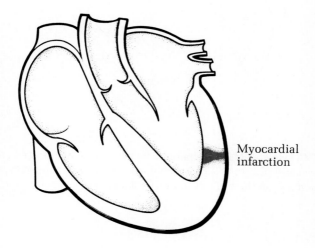

Myocardial
infarction

Myocardial infarction (MI) progresses acutely through ischemia and injury, which are reversible, to necrosis, which is not. The pathology is reflected by inverted T waves, elevated ST segments, and pathological Q waves in the ECG leads over the infarct. The leads on the wall opposite the infarct may exhibit "reciprocal" changes, that is, depressed ST segments, tall R waves, and tall T waves, which indicate more extensive pathology and higher mortality.

ECG characteristics

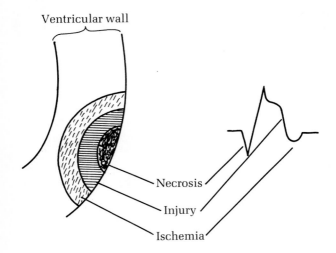

ECG signs of MI are supported by the clinical picture and an evolving picture as seen in serial tracings. The diagnosis never is made on the basis of the ECG alone.

Non–Q Wave Versus Q Wave MI

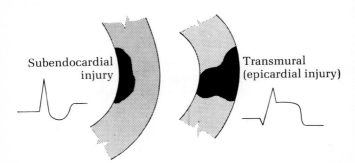

Q Wave MI

- Abnormal Q waves: Present
- ST segments: Elevated
- T waves: Deeply inverted, typically coved

Non–Q Wave MI

- Abnormal Q waves: None
- ST segments: Depressed
- T waves: Inverted in several limb and precordial leads

Diagnostic Leads

Type of infarct	Indicative changes (Q, ST elevation, T inversion)
Inferior	II, III, aV_F
Inferoposterior	II, III, aV_F, and reciprocal changes (precordial leads)
Septal	V_1 to V_2
Anterior wall	V_3 to V_4
Lateral wall	V_5 to V_6; I and aV_L
Posterior (acute)	V_1 to V_4 (reciprocal changes)
Right ventricular	ST elevation in V_{4R}

Acute Inferior Wall Infarction

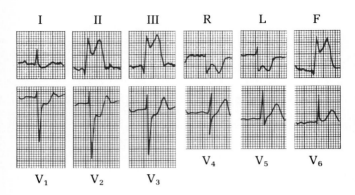

Inferoposterior MI

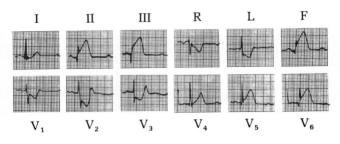

Inferoposterolateral MI

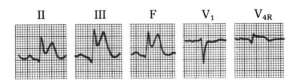

Inferior and right ventricular MI

ECG recognition of high risk

- Total ST elevation of more than 7 mm in leads II, III, and aV_F
- Reciprocal changes in the precordial leads (posterior and posteroseptal)
- ST elevation of more than 1 mm in lead V_{4R} (right ventricular MI)
- AV block

Acute Anterior Wall Infarction

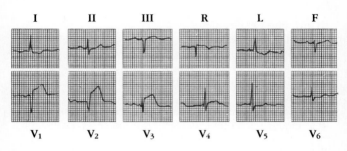

Anteroseptal MI

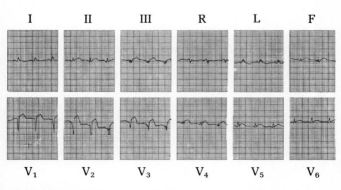

Anterolateral MI

ECG recognition of high risk

- Total ST elevation of more than 12 mm in precordial leads
- Presence of BBB and/or hemiblock

Identifying Candidates for Thrombolysis

Patients with large infarctions who receive therapy early after the onset of pain benefit the most from thrombolysis; small inferior infarctions usually do not require thrombolysis but are evaluated on an individual basis. Patients seen more than 6 hours from the onset of pain and the elderly may benefit also.

Absolute contraindications

- Active internal bleeding
- Suspected aortic dissection
- Recent head trauma or known intracranial neoplasm
- Diabetic hemorrhagic retinopathy
- Other hemorrhagic ophthalmic condition
- Pregnancy
- Previous allergic reaction to streptokinase or anisoylated plasminogen streptokinase activator complex (APSAC)*
  %Hypertension (> 200/120 mm Hg)
- History of cerebrovascular accident known to be hemorrhagic
- Trauma (including prolonged CPR) more recent than 2 weeks
- Major surgery within the past 2 months, especially intracranial or spinal surgery

---

*In the setting of previous allergic reaction to streptokinase or APSAC, either patients may be premedicated or, preferably, an alternative agent is used, such as tissue-type plasminogen activator (t-PA) or urokinase.

Relative contraindications (risk vs. benefit)

- Recent trauma or surgery (< 2 weeks)
- History of chronic severe hypertension with or without drug therapy
- Active peptic ulcer
- History of cerebrovascular accident
- Known predisposition to bleeding or current use of anticoagulants
- Significant liver dysfunction
- Prior exposure to streptokinase or APSAC (particularly important in the 6- to 9-month period after administration; applies to reuse of any streptokinase-containing agent but not to rt-PA or urokinase)

ECG Evaluation of Successful Reperfusion

- Continuous ST segment monitoring: the ST segment normalizes rapidly after reperfusion but remains unchanged with occlusion.
- Accelerated idioventricular rhythm: this arrhythmia is a sign of reperfusion.
- The QRS complex: reperfusion does not prevent development of Q waves, but their evolution accelerates, their sum is smaller, and some normalization occurs in the next 4 to 6 months.

Acute Pulmonary Embolism

14

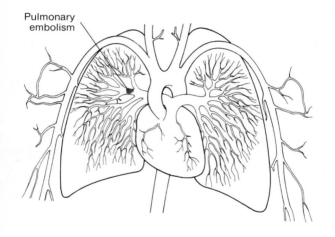

Pulmonary embolism

Accurate, rapid diagnosis and treatment are required in acute pulmonary embolism because it is often fatal and because early recognition and prompt treatment save the lives of at least 75% who would otherwise die. Although the ECG is not diagnostic of acute pulmonary embolism, common ECG findings raise suspicion and the diagnosis is confirmed by emergency echocardiogram.

Pathophysiology

Sudden obstruction of a central or peripheral pulmonary artery results in the following:

- Acute pulmonary hypertension
- Right-sided dilation
- Clockwise cardiac rotation
- Right ventricular failure
- Pulmonary infarction
- Marked ventilation/perfusion disturbance
- Acute lowering of the cardiac output

Signs and Symptoms

Physical findings are related to right ventricular hypertension, right ventricular failure, and the increase in pulmonary artery pressure. Physical findings are as follows:

- Tachypnea
- Dyspnea
- Sinus tachycardia
- Syncope
- Chest pain
- Cyanosis of the face
- Right ventricular heave
- Hepatomegaly
- Palpable right ventricular impulse
- Increase in jugular venous 'a' wave
- Increase in jugular venous distention
- Palpable pulmonary artery pulsation
- Tricuspid regurgitation
- Audible right ventricular S4
- S3 heart sound
- Narrow splitting of S2 with an exaggerated P2
- Pulmonary ejection murmur

Common ECG Findings

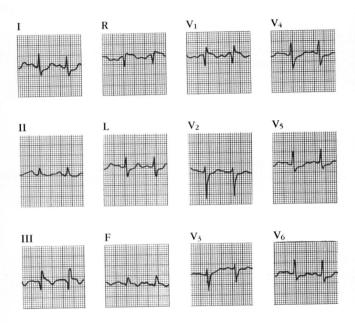

- RBBB
- S_1, Q_3, T_3
- Inverted T waves in V_2 and V_3
- Transitional zone shifts left
- ST elevation V_1, aV_R, III
- Frontal plane QRS axis shift to the right by 20 degrees or more
- P-pulmonale (P waves 2.5 mm in II, III, and aV_F)
- P wave right axis deviation
- Sinus tachycardia
- Atrial fibrillation
- Atrial flutter
- Premature beats (right atrial, right ventricular)
- Ventricular fibrillation

The Echocardiogram

Although pulmonary angiography remains the definitive technique for the diagnosis of pulmonary embolism, cardiac Doppler sonography from above the sternum offers a reliable alternative. The diagnosis is based on indirect signs of increased pressure in the pulmonary circulation, such as acute cor pulmonale with dilation of the right atrium and ventricle, central pulmonary vessels, and inferior vena cava.

Differential Diagnosis

Acute MI.

Treatment

1. Oxygen.
2. Analgesics.
3. Full-dose heparin.
4. Thrombolytic therapy.
5. Emergency pulmonary angiography and pulmonary embolectomy could be life saving in patients with acute massive pulmonary embolism.

Prevention

1. Anticoagulants.
2. Frequent change of body position.
3. Early ambulation.
4. When on complete bedrest, external compression of the legs.

Chamber Enlargement   15

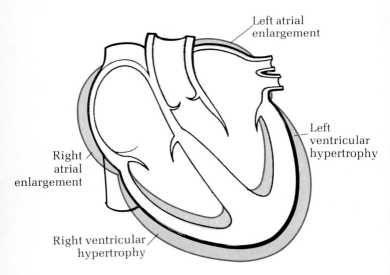

Left atrial enlargement

Left ventricular hypertrophy

Right atrial enlargement

Right ventricular hypertrophy

The term *chamber enlargement* refers to hypertrophy or dilation of the individual cardiac chambers and to the overall size of the heart. It indicates heart disease and is the mechanism by which the heart compensates for an increased load. It is usually the result of a chronic condition, such as valvular stenosis, which demands increased cardiac work and causes an actual increase in the size of muscular fibers. Indeed, an ECG finding of right ventricular hypertrophy (RVH) may be the first clue to the diagnosis of pulmonic stenosis; or left ventricular hypertrophy (LVH) may be the first sign of hypertrophic cardiomyopathy. The myocardium has the ability to increase its protein content by as much as 50% in response to such demands.

Left Ventricular Hypertrophy

Pathophysiology and mechanism

Increased QRS amplitude.   When the left ventricular wall hypertrophies, the disproportion in size between the left and right ventricles is increased, resulting in greater QRS amplitude, but a normal sequence of depolarization is retained (Figure 15-1).

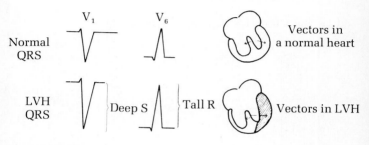

Figure 15-1
The normal QRS compared with that in LVH.

Intrinsicoid deflection.   This component of the QRS complex (the peak of the R wave) reflects the time it takes for peak voltage to develop under that particular electrode. Because there is more muscle mass, this deflection is delayed in V_6 (Figure 15-2).

Figure 15-2
The intrinsicoid deflection in V_6 in LVH.

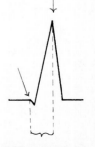

0.05 sec or more

Axis. The axis in LVH is normal because the conduction sequence is normal. As the heart hypertrophies, it rotates counterclockwise (posteriorly), producing a horizontal axis. A marked left axis shift suggests left anterior hemiblock, which may result from myocardial fibrosis secondary to longstanding hypertension.

"Strain" pattern. The mechanism is unknown, but it correlates with increasing left ventricular mass. It is known to be associated with longstanding LVH and to intensify when dilation and failure develop.

ECG characteristics (see also Table 15-1)

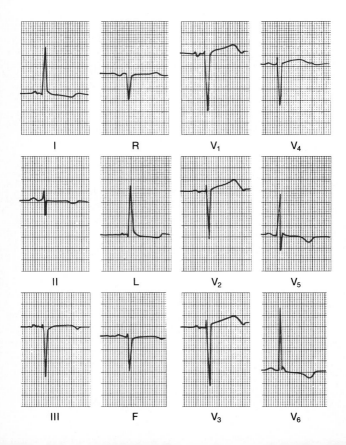

Table 15-1   Estes scoring system for left ventricular hypertrophy*

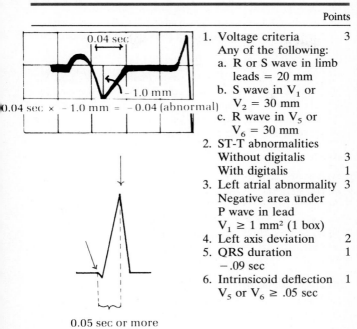

	Points

1. Voltage criteria
 Any of the following:
   a. R or S wave in limb leads = 20 mm
   b. S wave in V_1 or V_2 = 30 mm
   c. R wave in V_5 or V_6 = 30 mm
	3

2. ST-T abnormalities
   Without digitalis
   With digitalis
	3
	 1

3. Left atrial abnormality Negative area under P wave in lead $V_1 \geq 1$ mm^2 (1 box)	3
4. Left axis deviation	2
5. QRS duration $-.09$ sec	1
6. Intrinsicoid deflection V_5 or $V_6 \geq .05$ sec	1

*5 Points, diagnostic; 4 points, probable.

Note that the sensitivity of the ECG is limited in LVH

Rate.   Normal.

Rhythm.   Normal.

PR interval.   Normal.

QRS complex.   Increased amplitude; however, QRS voltage:

1. Varies with age (greater in the young)
2. Is normally greatest in the lead whose axis is parallel with the main current flow (electrical axis)
3. Is greater in individuals with a thin chest wall
4. Is less in obese individuals and in those with lung disease

Distinguishing features

1. Taller R waves in the left precordial leads.
2. Deeper S waves in the right precordial leads.
3. Intrinsicoid deflection delayed in V_6 to 0.05 sec or more (measured from the onset of the QRS to the peak of the R wave).
4. Axis is normal.
5. "Strain" pattern: ST-T-U abnormalities in V_5 and V_6. The ST segment is depressed with an upward convexity. The downward curve of the ST segment becomes an inverted T wave. U waves often invert.
6. Associated left atrial enlargement.

Causes

- Hypertension
- Aortic stenosis
- Aortic insufficiency
- Coarctation of the aorta
- Hypertrophic cardiomyopathy
- Athletics
- Myocardial infarction

Clinical implications

The ECG signs of cardiac enlargement or hypertrophy are not sensitive, although they are specific.

The patient care is supportive; the condition is a manifestation of another condition. There will be cardiac dysfunction because of increasing ventricular stiffness, elevated ventricular pressure, decreased passive ventricular filling, and decreased coronary blood flow, all of which will compound the seriousness should the patient sustain a myocardial infarction.

The patient may have a predisposition to subendocardial ischemia, and, if there is outflow tract obstruction, syncope frequently can occur because of an absent pressure gradient between the body of the left ventricle and the subaortic chamber.

Differential diagnosis

See "Causes."

Treatment

That of the primary disease.

Right Ventricular Hypertrophy

Pathophysiology and mechanism

Normally the electrical forces of the thicker left ventricle dominate those of the right ventricle so that an rS appears in V_1 and a qR in V_5 and V_6. In marked right ventricular hypertrophy the right ventricle dominates, there is right axis deviation, and the precordial pattern reverses (a tall R wave appears in V_1 and a deep S wave in V_6). A normal sequence of depolarization is retained (Figure 15-3).

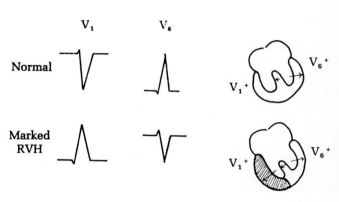

Figure 15-3
The normal QRS compared with that in RVH.

ECG characteristics

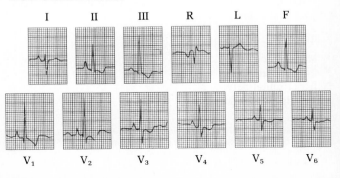

Rate.   Normal.

Rhythm.   Normal.

PR interval.   Normal.

QRS complex.   Normal, but Q waves may develop in II, III, and aV_F.

Distinguishing features

1. Right axis deviation of greater than +110 degrees in adults
2. Right axis deviation of greater than +120 degrees in the young
3. S_1, S_2, S_3 pattern in children
4. Late intrinsicoid deflection in V_1 and V_2
5. Incomplete right bundle branch block pattern in V_1 (rSr')
6. ST segment depression with upward convexity and inverted T waves in V_1 and V_2 and in the limb leads, with tall R waves
7. Reversal of precordial lead R wave progression
8. "Strain" patterns in V_1, V_2, II, III, and aV_F
9. Tall, peaked P waves in leads II, III, and aV_F and sometimes in V_1 (right atrial involvement)
10. Associated right atrial enlargement

Murphy has formulated two methods for identifying right ventricular hypertrophy*:

Method 1 (59% sensitivity, 86% specificity); positive if one of the following is present:

1. R/S ratio in V_5 or V_6 is 1.
2. S in V_5 or V_6 is 7 mm.
3. Right axis deviation of +90 degrees.
4. P-pulmonale.

Method 2 (40% sensitivity, 97% specificity); positive if any two of the above are present.

Causes

- Mitral stenosis
- Chronic lung disease
- Atrial septal defect
- Tetralogy of Fallot

*From Murphy ME et al: Reevaluation of electrocardiographic criteria for left, right, and combined cardiac ventricular hypertrophy, *Am J Cardiol* 53:1140, 1984.

- Pulmonary stenosis
- Tricuspid insufficiency

Clinical implications

The causes of right ventricular overload are not as common as the causes of left ventricular overload, and the fully developed ECG pattern is not often seen.

The nursing care is determined by the cause.

Rhythm variations

None.

Differential diagnosis

See "Causes."

Treatment

That of the primary disease.

Left Atrial Enlargement

Pathophysiology and mechanism

Same as for left ventricular hypertrophy.

ECG characteristics

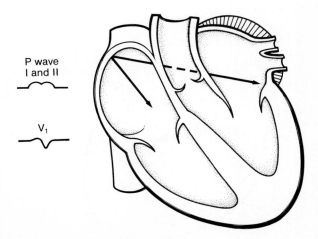

P wave
I and II

V_1

PR interval.   Normal.

QRS complex.   Often that of left ventricular hypertrophy.

Distinguishing features.   P wave (P-mitrale):
1. Widened to 0.12 sec or more
2. Notched with 0.04 sec between peaks
3. Deep, broad, negative terminal trough in V_1
4. May be negative in III and aV_F

Causes

■ Those of left ventricular hypertrophy

Pattern variations

None.

Differential diagnosis

None.

Treatment

That of the primary disease.

 Right Atrial Enlargement

Pathophysiology and mechanism

Same as for right ventricular hypertrophy.

ECG characteristics

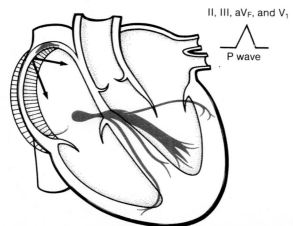

Rate. Normal.

Rhythm. Normal.

PR interval. Normal.

QRS complex. qR in V_1 in the absence of myocardial infarction; diminished voltage in V_1 with threefold or more increase in V_2.

Distinguishing features

1. Tall peaked P waves in II, III, and aV_F and sometimes in V_1 (P-pulmonale)
2. P wave axis to the right of $+70$ degrees (in chronic lung disease)

Causes

■ Those of right ventricular hypertrophy

Pattern variations

None.

Differential diagnosis

Left atrial enlargement. If the right atrium enlarges enough to extend toward the left, the P waves of right atrial enlargement may be inverted in V_1, simulating left atrial enlargement.

Treatment

That of the primary disease.

The Effects of Potassium and Calcium on the ECG

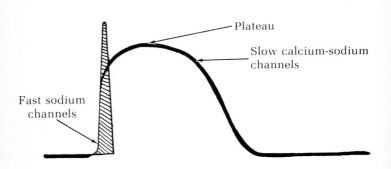

16

Plateau

Slow calcium-sodium channels

Fast sodium channels

ᙏᙏ Hyperkalemia

Pathophysiology and mechanism

Elevation of the serum potassium level decreases the resting membrane potential and causes conduction problems.

ECG characteristics

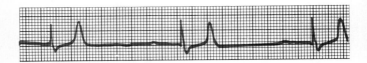

PR interval. Normal, but P wave disappears as level of potassium rises.

QRS complex. Widens.

Distinguishing features.   Tall, peaked T waves, loss of ST segment, left axis deviation, wide QRS, P wave of low amplitude or barely visible.

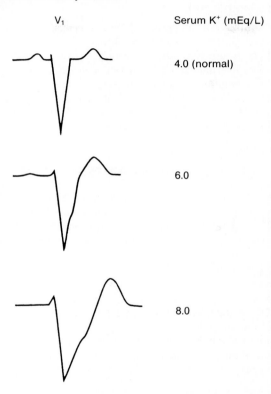

V₁   Serum K⁺ (mEq/L)

4.0 (normal)

6.0

8.0

5.5 mEq/L: T wave peaks; QRS widens; PR prolonged; P wave widens and becomes shallow

6.5 mEq/L: QRS widens more and shows marked slurring of second portion

8 mEq/L: QRS is slurred and wider; P wave is barely visible; S wave ascends directly into tall, peaked T wave; left axis deviation (QRS)

12 mEq/L: P wave disappears

Cause

■ Kidney failure (most common cause)

Clinical implications

This condition is potentially lethal but readily reversible; therefore early diagnosis is imperative.

There is no constant association between an absolute potassium level and the ECG; the rate of progression of cardiac toxicity is variable, and signs and symptoms are not uniformly present. Therefore maintain clinical suspicion, especially in patients with anoxia, acidosis, trauma to soft tissues, oliguria, or a history of spironolactone or triamterene ingestion.

Treatment

The choice of treatment depends on the severity of the hyperkalemia.

1. The patient is constantly monitored on the ECG.
2. Hypertonic Na^+ and Ca^{++} are indicated only if toxicity is advanced at time of discovery. They suppress the effects of hyperkalemia without affecting the potassium concentration.
3. Sodium bicarbonate in the presence of systemic acidosis lowers the serum potassium level by promoting cellular uptake.
4. Glucose and insulin promote uptake of potassium into liver and muscle cells.
5. Sorbitol and polystyrene sulfonate resin lower the total body potassium by cationic exchange.
6. Dialysis.

Hypokalemia

Pathophysiology and mechanism

At first hypokalemia causes an increase in the resting membrane potential (it becomes more negative), but this is soon followed by an increase in phase 4 depolarization in Purkinje fibers, which produces spontaneous ectopic beats and a resting maximal diastolic potential that becomes less and less negative until the fibers are nonexcitable. As the giant U wave appears, the patient is vulnerable to torsades de pointes.

ECG characteristics

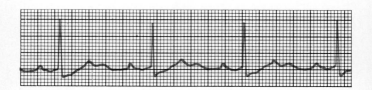

Rate.   Normal.

Rhythm.   Normal.

PR interval.   Lengthens slightly.

QRS complex.   Widens and amplitude increases (advanced stage).

Distinguishing features.   The U wave gets taller and taller and fuses with the T wave. There is progressive ST depression and decreased T wave amplitude.

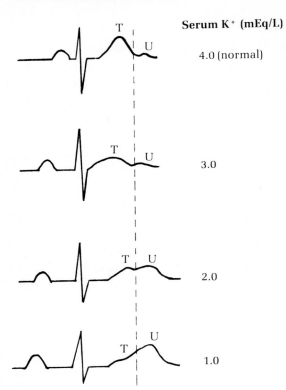

Serum K$^+$ (mEq/L)

4.0 (normal)

3.0

2.0

1.0

4 mEq/L: Normal U wave is same polarity as T wave and of low amplitude

3 mEq/L: T wave and U wave are same amplitude

2 mEq/L: U wave is taller than T wave

1 mEq/L: Giant U wave fuses with T wave

Causes

- Diuretics
- Vomiting
- Gastric suction

Clinical implications

The diagnosis is made because of the ECG picture, the symptoms of polyuria in mild cases, and muscle weakness in more severe cases. Hypokalemia may lead to torsades de pointes (p. 92).

In the patient taking digitalis even slight hypokalemia may precipitate serious arrhythmias.

Treatment

The route of repletion depends on the severity of the hypokalemia. The oral route is used in mild to moderate uncomplicated hypokalemia.

Hypercalcemia

Pathophysiology and mechanism

ECG changes resulting from changes in serum calcium levels are of clinical importance only when they are extremely high or low. Calcium exerts itself on the plateau of the action potential (phase 2). Thus the length of the QT interval is inversely related to serum calcium concentration: hypercalcemia shortens the QT interval.

ECG characteristics

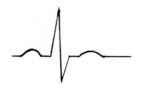

QT shortens

Rate.   Normal.
Rhythm.   Normal.
PR interval.   Normal.
QRS complex.   Normal.
Distinguishing features.   Short QT interval (not always a reliable sign).

Causes

- Malignancy
- Vitamin D intoxication
- Sarcoidosis
- Primary hyperparathyroidism
- Milk-alkali syndrome
- Thyrotoxicosis
- Adrenal insufficiency
- Vitamin A intoxication
- Idiopathic hypercalcemia in infants
- Immobilization
- Renal failure

 ## Clinical implications

Severe hypercalcemia is life threatening. If the patient is taking digitalis, intoxication may result.

Treatment

The cause is treated, and calcium excretion is promoted.

 # Hypocalcemia

Pathophysiology and mechanism

Because the length of the QT interval is inversely related to serum calcium concentration, hypocalcemia lengthens it. This lengthening of the refractory period as reflected in the QT interval is homogeneous, so that hypocalcemia rarely causes arrhythmias unless it is complicated by hypokalemia.

ECG characteristics

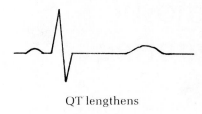

QT lengthens

Rate. Normal.
Rhythm. Normal.
PR interval. Normal.
QRS complex. Normal.
Distinguishing features. Long QT interval.

Causes

- Hypoparathyroidism
- Hypomalacia in adults and rickets in children
- Chronic steatorrhea
- Pregnancy
- Diuretics, such as furosemide or ethacrynic acid
- Respiratory alkalosis and hyperventilation
- Hypomagnesemia, possibly secondary to release of parathyroid hormone

Clinical implications

The cause of the deficiency must be identified and treated. A thorough history and physical examination are indicated.

Treatment

The cause is treated, and calcium is replaced.

Emergency Diagnostic Monitoring Leads

17

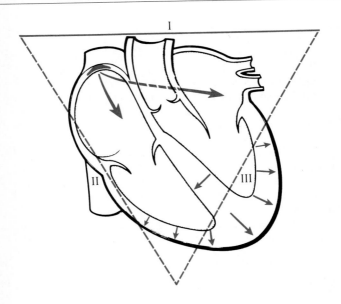

When a full 12-lead ECG is not immediately available, it is important to know which leads are mandatory for a diagnosis in the emergency setting.

 Paroxysmal Supraventricular Tachycardia

Minimal lead requirements. I, II, III, V_1, and V_6 during the tachycardia and after conversion to sinus rhythm.

Rationale.   To make the differential diagnosis between AV nodal reentry tachycardia and circus movement tachycardia using an accessory pathway, it is necessary to evaluate P′ wave location. P waves are small and sometimes are seen in one lead and not in another. The more leads recorded during the tachycardia, the better the chance of identifying P waves and the mechanism.

P waves often can be more easily spotted when a comparison is made of the QRS and ST segment during the two rhythms (tachycardia and sinus). In AV nodal reentry tachycardia, the P′ wave often distorts the QRS, whereas in circus movement tachycardia, the P′ wave usually distorts the ST segment, immediately following the QRS.

Digitalis Toxicity

Minimal lead requirements.   II and V_1.

Rationale.   Patients taking digitalis glycosides are monitored in lead II if P waves are present and in lead V_1 if there is atrial fibrillation. The atrial tachycardia caused by digitalis toxicity has upright P waves in lead II, very similar in shape to the sinus P wave. Once the atrial rhythm has been evaluated, one looks for AV dissociation. If it is present or if there are no P waves, as in atrial fibrillation, the best lead to evaluate is V_1. In this lead a junctional or a fascicular rhythm can be discerned because of the shape of the ventricular complex. The shape of the QRS in a junctional rhythm will be that of the normal QRS (rS); the fascicular rhythm looks like right bundle branch block (rSR′).

Wide Complex Tachycardia

Minimal lead requirements. V_1 often suffices; occasionally V_2 and V_6 are required.

Rationale.   When the ventricular complex in V_1 is positive, a monophasic, biphasic, or Rr′ pattern indicates VT. In the case of an rR′ pattern, V_6 is necessary; an R : S ratio of less than 1 in that lead indicates VT.

When the ventricular complex in V_1 is negative, V_1 and V_2 are evaluated for signs of VT: an R wave > 0.03 sec, a slurred S downstroke, or an S nadir delayed more than 0.06 sec. A Q wave in V_6 also is indicative of VT.

Unstable Angina

Minimal lead requirements. V_2 and V_3 when pain-free; 12 leads during pain.

Rationale. During the pain-free period of unstable angina, a progressively inverting, symmetrical T wave in leads V_2 and V_3 without loss of precordial R wave and with little or no CK elevation indicates critical proximal left anterior descending coronary artery occlusion.

During the pain of unstable angina, a 12-lead ECG is obtained to evaluate for left mainstem or three-vessel disease, indicated by ST elevation in leads aV_R and V_1 and ST depression in approximately 8 other leads.

High-Risk Myocardial Infarction

Minimal lead requirements. A 12-lead ECG is of course needed for the diagnosis of myocardial infarction. For assessment of high risk in acute inferior wall infarction, lead V_{4R} also is necessary. For assessment of high risk in acute anterior wall infarction, leads V_1, I, and II are necessary.

Rationale. In acute inferior wall infarction, the development of an elevated ST segment in the right chest lead, V_{4R}, indicates proximal right coronary artery occlusion, right ventricular infarction, a higher incidence of AV block, and greater risk. Other ECG signs of high risk are ST depression in the precordial leads and high-grade AV block.

In acute anterior wall infarction, the development of RBBB and/or hemiblock indicates high risk. RBBB is diagnosed in lead V_1, and the axis deviation of hemiblock is seen in leads I and II.

Pacemaker Therapy for Bradycardia 18

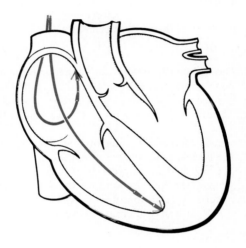

Electronic pacemakers can repetitively stimulate cardiac muscle and are the principle therapy for symptomatic patients with bradycardia. All pacing systems are capable of directly pacing the ventricular muscle (single-chamber pacemaker). In patients with reliable AV conduction, pacing of the atrial muscle alone (single-chamber pacemaker) is an option also. AV pacemakers are capable of stimulating both the atria and the ventricles (dual-chamber pacemaker).

The Pacing System

The pacing system consists of a pulse generator and a lead electrode. The pulse generator contains the pacemaker electronics and the energy source for generating electrical stimuli.

The lead electrode, which may be unipolar or bipolar, is attached by a wire to the pulse generator and makes contact with the cardiac tissue to conduct the stimuli from the pulse generator.

Sensing

The sensing feature prevents delivery of stimuli to refractory muscle by sensing natural depolarizations and using this information to control timing. The term *undersensing* refers to the rare occasions when a depolarization is not sensed. This may occur with a nonuniform ectopic depolarization. *Oversensing* refers to the sensing of interference.

Timing

Pacemakers continuously monitor the timing between natural or paced depolarizations and compare them with the ones stored in the pulse generator. If an impulse fails to occur within an expected time, the pacemaker sends a stimulus to the muscle.

The pacemaker intercycle timing may be A-A, in which the atrial impulse is used to set the time limit for the appearance of the atrial event of the next cycle. In V-V cycle timing, the ventricular event sets the time limit for the start of the next ventricular event. An atrioventricular (AV) pacemaker may use A-A or V-V, or it may alternate between them.

Magnet Mode

Almost all pacemakers contain a switch that when activated by a magnet suspends sensing so that the pacing function can be observed. This is necessary when a pacemaker is inhibited by natural depolarizations.

Five-Letter Pacemaker Code

The five-position pacemaker code of the Intersociety Committee on Heart Disease (ICHD) is used universally to describe pacemaker operation; the first three positions are used most often. The first four letters apply to pacing bradycardias; a fifth letter (not shown here) is used for antitachycardia pacing.

Pacemaker Modes (Four-Letter Code)

1	2	3	4
Chamber Paced	Chamber Sensed	Mode of Response	Features
V = Ventricle	V = Ventricle	I = Inhibits pacing	P = Programmable
A = Atrium	A = Atrium	T = Triggered	M = Multiprogrammable
D = Dual chamber	D = Dual chamber	D = Dual (Both I and T)	C = Communicating
S = Single chamber	S = Single chamber	0 = None	R = Rate modulating

Responsive Heart Rate Pacemakers

Pacemakers can automatically vary their rate to match the needs of the patient. If the patient has a naturally responsive atrial rate, the pacemaker can track this natural activity and synchronize the ventricles with it. If the patient does not have a naturally responsive atrial rate, the pacemaker monitors other parameters that correlate with cardiovascular activity, such as activity, respiration, neurohumoral drive, and blood pressure, to determine the desired pacing rate.

The pacemaker will never pace slower than the programmable lower rate limit (PLRL) nor faster than the programmable upper rate limit (PURL).

Clinical Application

Atrial bradycardia with reliable AV conduction

AAIR (atrial demand pacing with rate modulation). It is necessary to pace and sense only in the atria, since AV conduction is good. Atrial sensing inhibits any natural atrial activity. A responsive heart rate is provided with the added feature of rate modulation.

Good atrial rhythm with unreliable AV conduction

DDD (universal atrioventricular pacing). The atria's own responsive heart rate is used to pace the ventricles (AV synchrony). The ventricles are also sensed and inhibited to prevent competition should natural AV conduction take place.

Intermittent atrial bradycardia with unreliable AV conduction

DDDR (rate-modulated universal atrioventricular pacing). Again the ventricles must be paced, sensed, and inhibited for the same reasons just mentioned. With the unreliable atrial rhythm, a sensor is used to ensure a responsive heart rate.

Constant atrial bradycardia with unreliable AV conduction

DVIR (rate-modulated AV sequential pacing). The pacemaker must pace the atria and trigger an AV interval to synchronize the ventricular pacing. The ventricles are paced and sensed.

Atrial fibrillation with unreliable conduction

VVIR (ventricular-inhibited demand mode with rate modulation). The best scenario here is that the ventricles be paced and sensed and that the rate be modulated with a sensor.

AAI Pacing

II

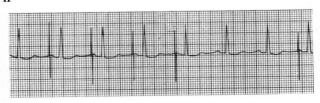

In the AAI mode, pacing and sensing occur only in the atrium and the pacemaker is inhibited by sensed atrial activity. This type of pacemaker is appropriate only when AV conduction is adequate.

VDD Pacing

II

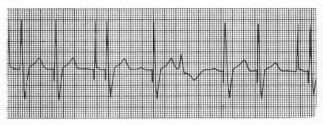

In VDD pacing, atrial activity is sensed and the ventricle is paced in synchrony. Pacing occurs only in the ventricle, but sensing occurs in both chambers. The pacemaker is triggered by intrinsic atrial activity and inhibited by intrinsic ventricular activity. If the intrinsic atrial rate falls below the programmed ventricular rate, only the ventricle will be paced. In such a case the pacemaker functions in the VVI mode. Such pacing is appropriate when AV conduction is not intact and ventricular pacing is necessary.

DVI Pacing

V₁

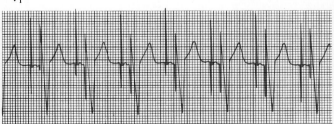

The DVI mode is dual-chamber pacing. Pacing occurs in either the atrium or the ventricle, or in both, but sensing occurs only in the ventricle. The pacemaker is inhibited by intrinsic ventricular activity.

DDD Pacing

V_1

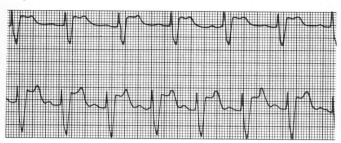

The DDD mode provides another form of dual-chamber pacing; pacing and sensing occur in either the atrium or the ventricle, or in both. Atrial or ventricular output is inhibited by sensed atrial or ventricular activity, and ventricular output is triggered by sensed atrial activity.

The DDD pacemaker has the potential to operate in four modes (VVI, AAI, VDD, and DVI), adapting to the patient's rhythm. Such a pacemaker is totally inhibited by the patient's normal sinus rhythm. However, if there is sinus bradycardia, it paces the atrium (AAI); if there is prolonged or blocked atrioventricular (AV) conduction, it paces both the atrium and the ventricle sequentially (DDD).

The Pacemaker Syndrome

The pacemaker syndrome is weakness or syncope related to adverse hemodynamic effects of ventricular pacing. The causes are loss of atrial kick and simultaneous atrial and ventricular contraction.

Indications for Permanent Cardiac Pacemaker Implantation

Permanent cardiac pacemaker implantation in the treatment of bradyarrhythmias is justified, even if the patient is asymptomatic, when the AV block is at the level of the bundle branches and manifesting as type II second-degree or complete AV block.

In all other clinical settings the following conditions are met before permanent pacing can be instituted:

- Drugs must be excluded as a cause of conduction or impulse generation problems.
- The patient must be experiencing serious symptoms as a result of failure of impulse generation or conduction.

Indications for Temporary Pacing

Indications for temporary pacing include the following:

- After open heart surgery
- During cardiac catheterization or surgery
- Before implantation of permanent pacemaker
- Anterior wall myocardial infarction with right bundle branch block and left anterior hemiblock or concurrent left bundle branch block
- Acute inferior myocardial infarction with refractory complete AV block and ventricular ectopics, hemodynamic deterioration, or both
- Termination of atrial flutter, paroxysmal supraventricular tachycardia, or ventricular tachycardia
- Electrophysiologic studies

Endocardial Puncture

Endocardial puncture results in cessation of pacing. If the patient is taking anticoagulants, cardiac tamponade may result. Endocardial puncture is confirmed by obtaining a unipolar electrogram from the distal electrode. This is done by connecting the V lead to the tip electrode (cathode). If the electrode is situated in the right ventricular apex, the QRS complex is negative and the ST segment elevated (Figure 18-1, A). If the endocardium has been perforated and the electrode is within the pericardial sac, the QRS is positive, the ST segment depressed, and the T wave inverted (Figure 18-1, B).

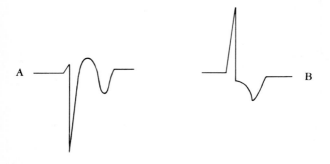

Figure 18-1
A, Pattern when the electrode is in the right ventricular apex. **B**, Pattern when the electrode has perforated the myocardium and is in the pericardial sac.

Pacemaker-Mediated Tachycardia

V_1

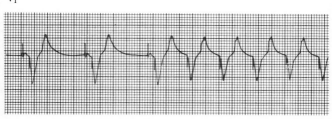

Pacemaker-mediated tachycardia is initiated when a retrograde P wave is sensed by a dual-chamber pacemaker, which in turn activates the ventricular pacemaker. If there is retrograde conduction from each ventricular beat and if the retrograde P wave reaches the atrium after the atrial refractory period and the pacemaker ventricular refractory period, an endless-loop tachycardia ensues. This may be avoided by programming an adequate atrial refractory period. In this way the retrograde P wave is not sensed.

One way to terminate such a tachycardia is to switch to a DVI mode, thus eliminating atrial sensing.

Evaluating a DDD Tracing
Evaluate the Atrial Event

1. Is a P wave present?
2. Is it paced or intrinsic?
3. What is the rate of the atrial event?

Evaluate AV Delay

The AV delay is programmable and is the time between atrial and ventricular activity during which the pacemaker is "looking for" an R wave.
1. Is there a programmed AV delay?
2. What is its value?
3. Is it the same as in the tracing?

Evaluate the Ventricular Event

1. Are there intrinsic or paced ventricular complexes?
2. At what rate?
3. Has intrinsic ventricular activity been sensed?

Evaluate the VA Interval

The VA interval is determined by subtracting the AV delay from the programmed pulse interval. During part of this time, sensing for atrial activity takes place. This interval is functioning normally if intrinsic ventricular activity resets the VA interval.

Index